Gold Standard Tec
Total Laparoscopic Hysterectomy

Gold Standard Technique of Total Laparoscopic Hysterectomy

Mehul V Sukhadiya MBBS DGO
Medical Director
Radhe Endoscopy Training Centre
Mehsana, Gujarat, India

Foreword
Gopal Hirani

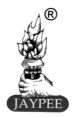

JAYPEE BROTHERS MEDICAL PUBLISHERS (P) LTD
New Delhi • London • Philadelphia • Panama

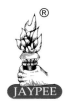

Jaypee Brothers Medical Publishers (P) Ltd.

Headquarters
Jaypee Brothers Medical Publishers (P) Ltd.
4838/24, Ansari Road, Daryaganj
New Delhi 110 002, India
Phone: +91-11-43574357
Fax: +91-11-43574314
Email: jaypee@jaypeebrothers.com

Overseas Offices

J.P. Medical Ltd.
83, Victoria Street, London
SW1H 0HW (UK)
Phone: +44-2031708910
Fax: +02-03-0086180
Email: info@jpmedpub.com

Jaypee-Highlights Medical Publishers Inc.
City of Knowledge, Bld. 237, Clayton
Panama City, Panama
Phone: +1 507-301-0496
Fax: +1 507-301-0499
Email: cservice@jphmedical.com

Jaypee Medical Inc.
The Bourse
111, South Independence Mall East
Suite 835, Philadelphia, PA 19106, USA
Phone: +1 267-519-9789
Email: jpmed.us@gmail.com

Jaypee Brothers Medical Publishers (P) Ltd.
17/1-B, Babar Road, Block-B, Shaymali
Mohammadpur, Dhaka-1207
Bangladesh
Mobile: +08801912003485
Email: jaypeedhaka@gmail.com

Jaypee Brothers Medical Publishers (P) Ltd.
Bhotahity, Kathmandu, Nepal
Phone: +977-9741283608
Email: kathmandu@jaypeebrothers.com

Website: www.jaypeebrothers.com
Website: www.jaypeedigital.com

© 2014, Jaypee Brothers Medical Publishers

The views and opinions expressed in this book are solely those of the original contributor(s)/author(s) and do not necessarily represent those of editor(s) of the book.

Inquiries for bulk sales may be solicited at: jaypee@jaypeebrothers.com

Gold Standard Technique of Total Laparoscopic Hysterectomy

First Edition: **2014**

ISBN: 978-93-5090-439-8

Printed at : Samrat Offset Pvt. Ltd.

Dedicated to

Lord Shree Swaminarayana Bhagvan
My Loving Family
and My Parents

Foreword

It gives me a great pleasure to write the foreword for *Gold Standard Technique of Total Laparoscopic Hysterectomy*. I am delighted that Dr Mehul V Sukhadiya is going to publish atlas about his refined bloodless technique of Total Laparoscopic Hysterectomy (TLH). I can definitely say that his technique is the Gold Standard. Myself is the witness of so many impossible difficult surgeries, which he simplifies by using Ruby bipolar and his own fabricated manipulator.

This atlas contains 500 colorful pictures from starting to last step, highlighting even likely complicated cases and how it has to be managed in present scenario. This atlas helps a lot during the day-to-day work such as ready-reckoner regarding query or solution in the learning stage of beginners.

I wish to all beginners, who are enthusiastic to learn Laparoscopic Hysterectomy that this atlas will be very useful, if its steps are followed to strengthen the confidence during endoscopy.

Dr Sukhdia's vast knowledge and experience has enlighten our motivation to do endoscopic surgery. In present scenario, I can say that his technique is compulsion to move every gynecologist to accept this modality of technique in future. Endoscopy has all solution of different diseases with excellent postoperative recovery and scarless abdomen. I am sure that readers will find this atlas very informative and useful.

Gopal Hirani MD (Gynec)
Senior Gynecologist
Hirani Maternity home
Bhuj, Gujarat, India

In today's high-tech era, everyone wants minimum pain and maximum recovery in shorter time. This thing only happens with Laparoscopy procedure.

Hysterectomy is the most common surgery in our day-to-day practice. When I was in learning phase, at that time I have attended so many workshops and conferences, and try to learn the technique of Total Laparoscopic Hysterectomy (TLH). I encountered many problems during the learning phase, therefore, I decided to develop very simple, safe and unique technique of TLH.

My technique of TLH is very simple, safe, easy, bloodless, reproducible and stepwise. This technique requires minimum instruments, staff; less time and pain; and less anesthesia. This technique is easily understood by the learner and after proper training anybody can perform it.

In this atlas, I have covered all aspects of hysterectomy, such as how to start and what are the precautions you should take during surgery to prevent bowel, bladder and ureteric injuries. This atlas contains 500 colorful pictures, procedure of TLH, how to prevent complications, how to manage difficult cases and also discuss about general anesthesia.

This atlas is really helpful for the student, gynecologist, surgeon and to whomever interested in TLH. It changes your ideas and views and removes unnecessary fear of laparoscopy.

Mehul V Sukhadiya

Acknowledgments

My special thanks to Dr Kirtiben Patel, Surat, Gujarat, India, for encouraging me to prepare atlas. My Laparoscopy teacher Dr Prakash Trivadi and other doctors, who supported me directly or indirectly, viz. Dr Pragnesh Shah, Dr Sanjay Patel, Dr HR Patel and Dr Pravin Patel. I am thankful to my Radhe Endoscopy Training Team, Anesthesia Team and Computer Operators— Mr Dilip Patel, Mr Mayank Sukhadiya and Mr Dash.

I acknowledge to Shri Jitendar P Vij (Group Chairman), Mr Ankit Vij (Managing Director), Mr Tarun Duneja (Director-Publishing), Mr KK Raman (Production Manager) Mr Neelambar Pant (Production Coordinator), Mr Sunil Kumar Dogra (Production Executive), Mr Manish Kumar Jha (Proofreader), Mr Varun Rana (Typesetter) and Mr Pawan Kumar (Graphic Designer) of M/s Jaypee Brothers Medical Publishers (P) Ltd, New Delhi, India, for their untiring efforts in the publication.

Contents

CHAPTER
1

Introduction

Gold Standard Technique of Total Laparoscopic Hysterectomy is Developed by Dr Sukhadiya

Hysterectomy is one of the most common surgeries in our day to day practice. Hysterectomy can be abdominal, vaginal, none descends vaginal, laparoscopic-assisted vaginal hysterectomy (LAVH) and total laparoscopic hysterectomy (TLH). Indeed, very good skill and technology, every surgery have some complication. Among them, TLH is good I do not go in detail, as all know about TLH real advantage. However, our technique is very simple, easy and low budget. Moreover, least complicating.

After so many changes, I developed this technique. It is very easy to learn and understand by our colleague and friends. You need proper laparoscopy training and understanding of basics principle of laparoscopy. You have to understand the way of using electrocautary machine, principle of surgery, maintanence of Instruments, mechanical aspects of equipments and other alternative. That can be learn From training centre, so I have FOGSI Recognized Radhe Endoscopy Training Centre. In our Centre we train our candidate in proper methodical way so they motivated for Laparoscopy surgery and start without fear.

CHAPTER
2

Why this Technique Consider Gold Standard?

Although, now a days so many techniques for TLH like without manipulation, direct uterine approach, two ports, one sided two ports, With harmonic use of robots and single port and so on.

Dr Sukhadiya's technique considers GOLD Standard and needy because-

- Very easy to learn and practically applicable
- Use of simple and basic instruments
- Minimum assistance only 2 required
- Minimum blood loose (Blood less)
- Minimal time
- Patient, needs fewer anesthesia
- **Patient can walk from Operation theater table**
- Fast recovery
- It is real cosmetic surgery
- Hour care only required
- Low Budge Surgery
- Least maintenance
- Maintaining of all surgical principal of hysterectomy
- Beginner and average gynecologist can do such type of surgery after training
- Without any problems
- Any Gynecologist performed AH, VH, LSCS, TL, D and C and other routine surgery same way they can perform TLH without fear.

CHAPTER 3

Instrument Required for Total Laparoscopic Hysterectomy

a. **Equipment:** Good quality of camera, single chip or three chips
   - Monitor
   - CO_2 insufflator
   - Light source and cable
   - Stabilizer.

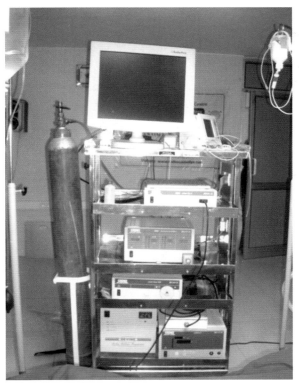

FIGURE 3.1: Laparoscopy trolley

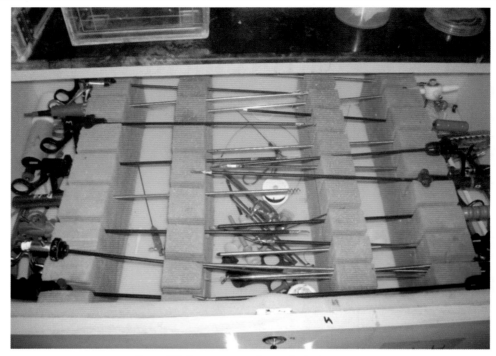

FIGURE 3.2: Laparoscopy drover for instruments

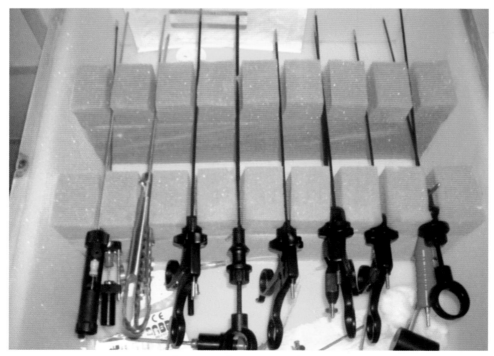

FIGURE 3.3: Three mm set drover

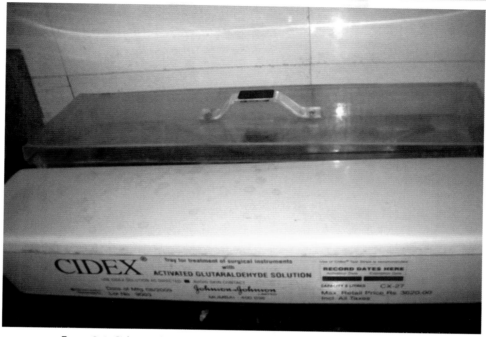

FIGURE 3.4: Cidex and saline tray for instruments sterilization and cleaning

b. ***Instrument:***
  1. *Optics:*
     - 10 mm 30-degree telescope
     - 5 mm 30-degree telescope.

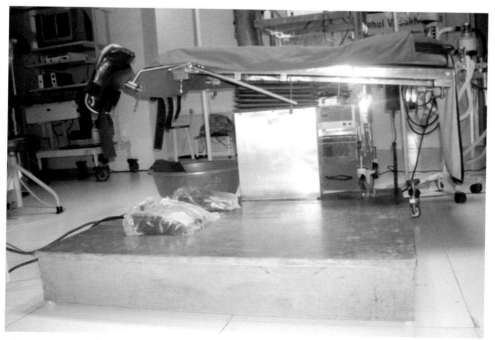

FIGURE 3.5: The remote control operation theater table with wooden platform for surgeon to stand. They are required for proper height therefore, patient abdomen at or below waist of surgeon and no shoulder pain, when work on right side

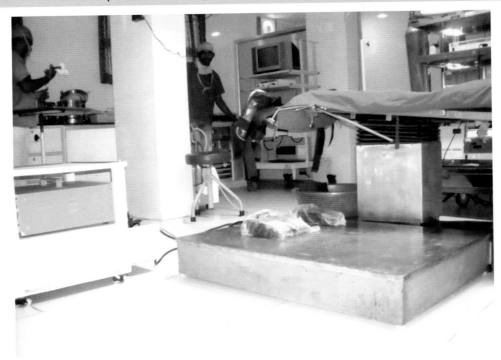

FIGURE 3.6: Always electrocautery unit away from laparoscopy trolley

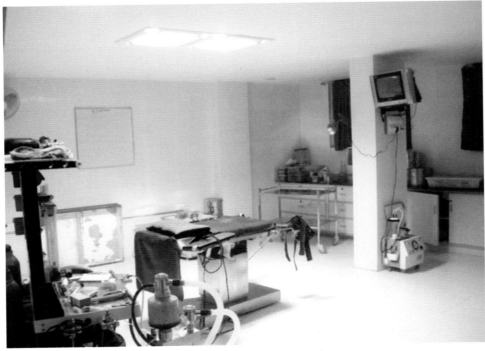

FIGURE 3.7: Spacious operation theater required in laparoscopy surgery

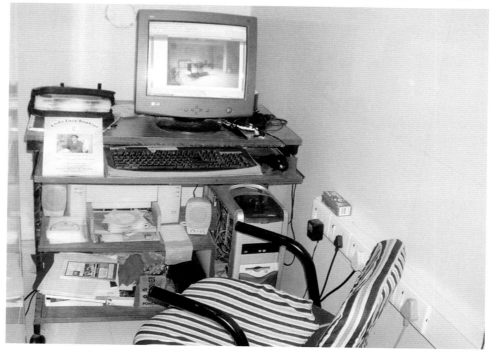

FIGURE 3.8: Separate video recording computer unit

2. *Trocars:*
   - 10 mm metal (1 or 2 require)
   - 5 mm plastic or metal (3 or 4 require)

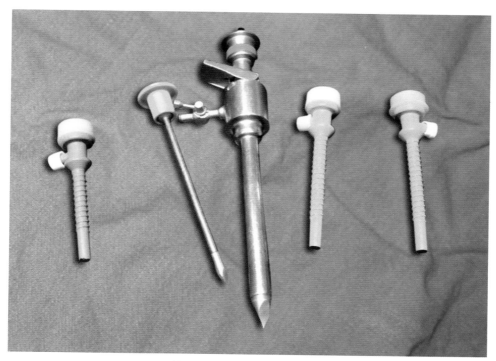

FIGURE 3.9: Trocar and Cannula

3. *Hand instruments*
    - Bipolar forceps
    - Curve scissor
    - Babcock forceps
    - Maryland forceps
    - Suction and irrigation
    - Needle holder
    - Tooth grasper with serration
    - Monopolar hook or spatula.

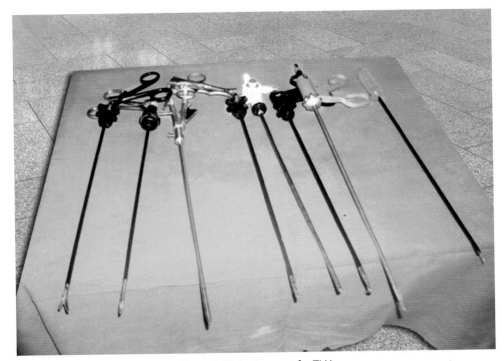

FIGURE 3.10: Instrument for TLH

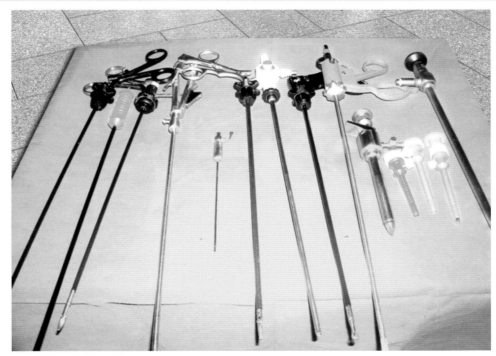

Figure 3.11: Total laparoscopic hysterectomy trolley

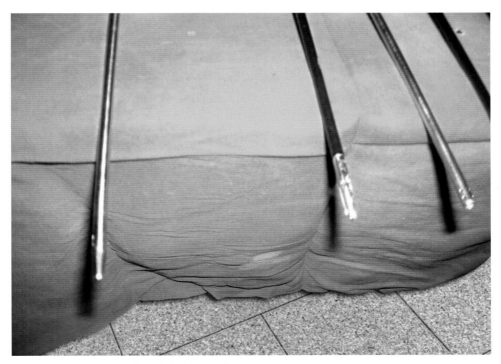

Figure 3.12: Needle holder, tooth serrated grasper and suction irrigation

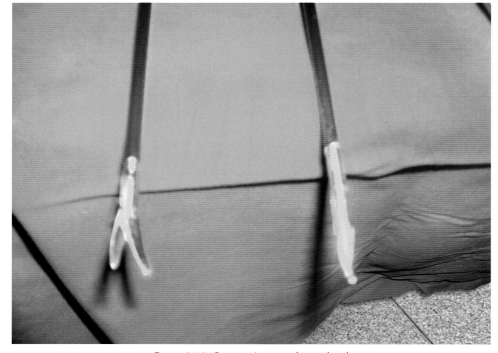

FIGURE 3.13: Curve scissor and maryland

4. *Electrocautery machine*

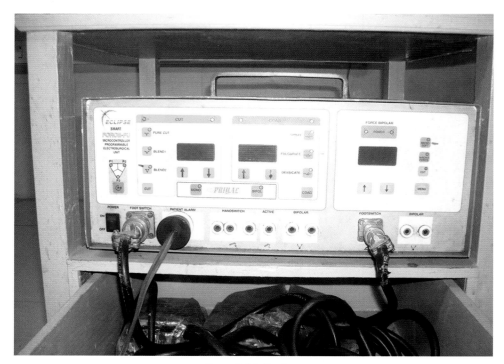

FIGURE 3.14: Cautery

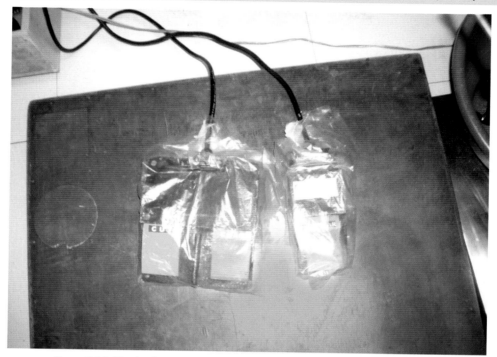

FIGURE 3.15: Bipolar foot switch 1st then monopolar foot switch that is routine

5. *Manipulator—Sukhadiya Manipulator*

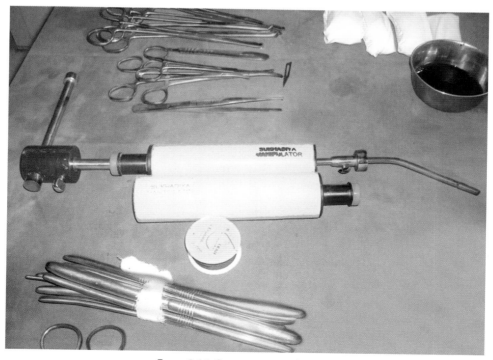

FIGURE 3.16: Separate vaginal trolley

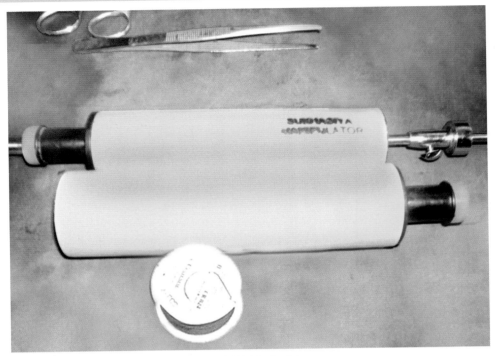

FIGURE 3.17: Manipulator

CHAPTER

4

Steps of this Technique

- After taking all preoperative steps patient taken in Operation Theater.
- Anesthetist always give general anesthesia to all posted for Laparoscopic surgery. Give proper position to patient her left hand should under same buttock, so that surgeon-getting good free space.
- **First** step is creation of pneumoperitoneum.
- I prefer open assess method for primary port. In this, I should open vertically umbilical tube (cutting of skin and sheath) very thinnest area to enter in abdominal cavity.
- **Second** step is use of three secondary ports under vision. First left lower port at just two finger medial and two finger above the anterior superior iliac spine (ASIS), second at midway between pubic symphysis and Umbilicus but 1 to 1.5 cm towards

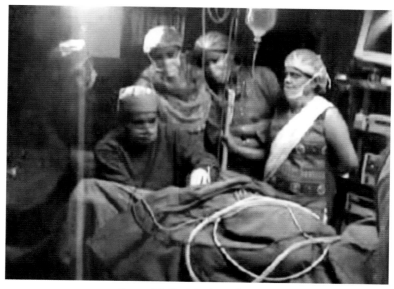

FIGURE **4.1:** Positioning of patient

left side and 3rd right lower port at just two finger medial and two finger above the ASIS. So, all three in same line but always above the fundus of uterus.

- Position of the primary and secondary port may change according to the size of uterus.
- **Third** step is examination of anatomy and other pathology account of ureteric path.
- Any adhesion remove 1st if possible, making normal anatomy then start Total Laparoscopic Hysterectomy
- **Fourth step:**
  - Keep everything ready before starting.
  - There are three steps of coagulation proximal, distal and middle of the stump.
  - Sign of coagulation is change of tissue color red-white-yellow then stop, if you do more coagulation, then it become dark charring effect start.
  - Other sign of coagulation is stoppage of bubbles.
- **Fifth step**
  - From left lower port introduce bipolar and from middle port scissors.
  - Starting from left cornual site, fallopian tube, ovarian ligament, round ligament and lastly ovarian vessels. About 1-1.5 cm away from cornu so bleeding becomes less.
- **Sixth step**
  - Then opening of two layers of broad ligament respectively posterior and anterior leaves.
  - For bladder dissection, just lift of UV fold of peritoneum and dissection with bipolar and scissor. In addition, dissection of bladder pillars so, no need of extra step for bladder dissection.
- **Seventh step**
  - Skeletonization of left uterine vessels then go for coagulation and cut.
- **Eighth step**
  - Then coagulation and cutting of cardinal and utero sacral ligament.
  - So, one-sided dissection is over.
- **Ninth step**
  - Still no change of instrument and proceed for right cornual dissection namely fallopian tube, ovarian ligament, round ligament and ovarian vessels.
  - Then change of only bipolar from left lower port to right lower port.
  - And same way proceeds for dissection of both leaves of broad ligament, skeletonization of uterine vessels, cardinal and utero sacral ligament.
  - Only remain part is vault of vagina.
- **Tenth step**
  - For vault dissection, pushes of vaginal tube in such a way that vault become prominent.
  - I use bipolar and monopolar for vault dissection.
  - I use more bipolar than monopolar at vault so, minimum spread of current.
  - Complete detachment of uterus from its attachment removed vaginally if, size is more, then need of morcellator for debulking.
  - Check for homeostasis.
  - Start suturing of vault with intracorporeal (contralateral or unilateral) technique whichever suitable to you. Nevertheless, contralateral is easy and simple technique.
  - For suturing, I use needle holder in left lower port and single teeth grasper with serration in right lower port.
  - I always prefer to use 45 cm suture material and 40 mm round body needle.
  - First taking left angle stitch and then taking some part of vault
  - Then right angle stitch with some part of vault of vagina so, no need of extra vault stitch
  - With each angle, stitch must take utero -sacral so, it maintains good vault support.
  - Use specimen at below for maintainance of pneumoperitoneum.
  - Remove needle with thread under vision.
  - At the end, do through lavage with saline.
  - At the end, check all pedicles without pneumo (means at 0 mm of Hg pressure).
  - Use same thread for closer of 10 mm port.

Keep everything ready before starting.

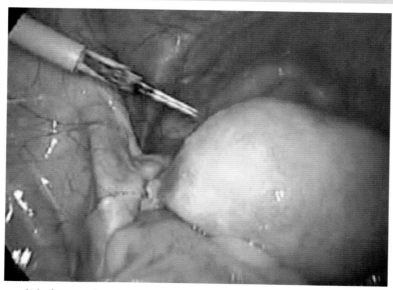

FIGURE 4.2: Keep everything ready before starting. First step is examination of anatomy and other pathology account of ureteric path

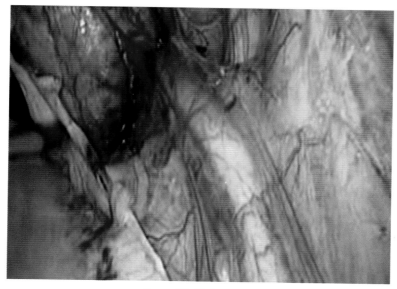

FIGURE 4.3: Right ureter

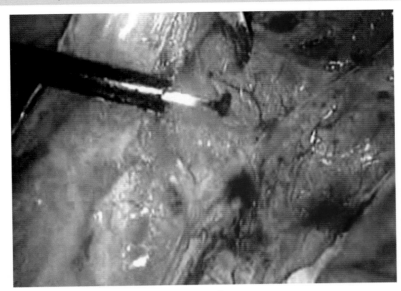

FIGURE 4.4: Left ureter

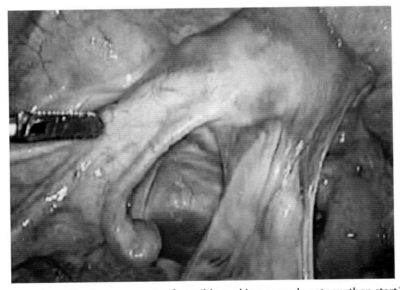

FIGURE 4.5: Any adhesion remove 1st if possible, making normal anatomy then start TLH

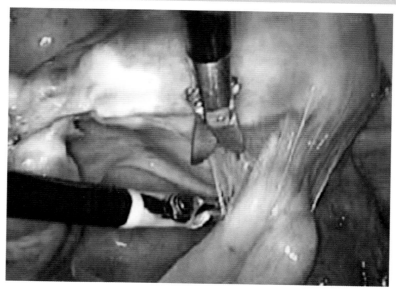

FIGURE **4.6:** Adhesiolysis

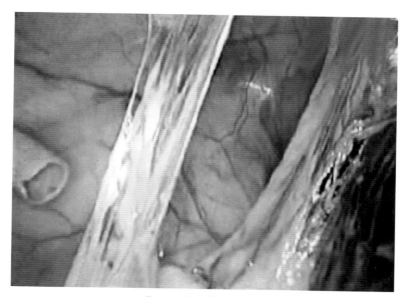

FIGURE **4.7:** Adhesiolysis

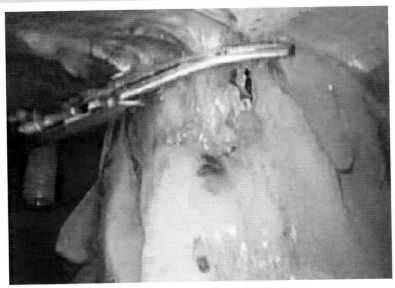

FIGURE **4.8:** Sharp dissection

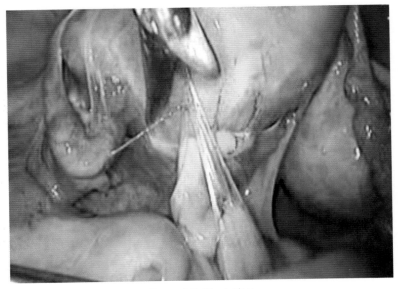

FIGURE **4.9:** Dissection

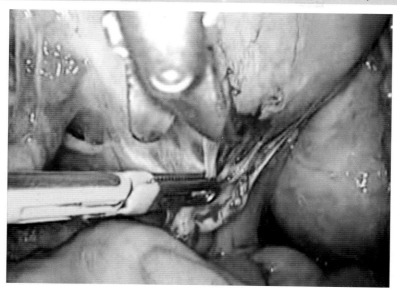

FIGURE **4.10:** Dissection flush to uterus

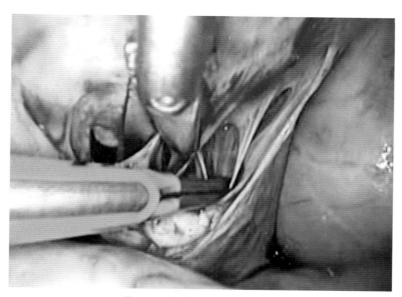

FIGURE **4.11:** Rectum dissection

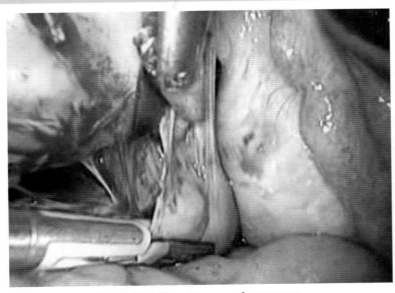

FIGURE 4.12: Dissection away from rectum

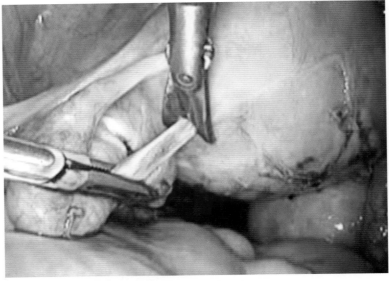

FIGURE 4.13: Adhesion band remove

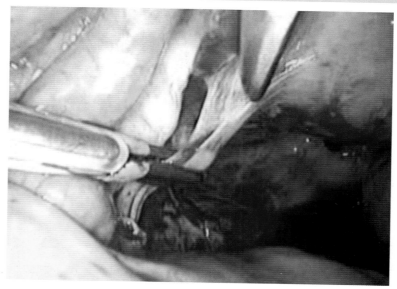

FIGURE 4.14: Adhesion removes

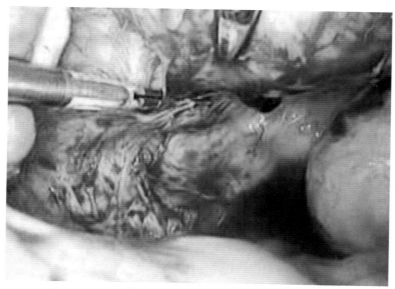

FIGURE 4.15: Complete adhesiolysis, then start main surgery

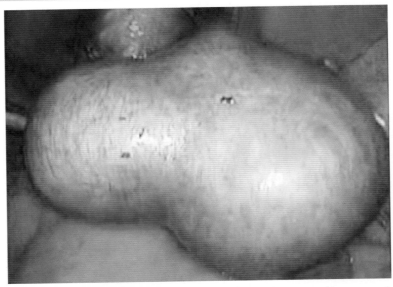

FIGURE 4.16: Size does not matter up to 32 weeks size uterus removed laparoscopically

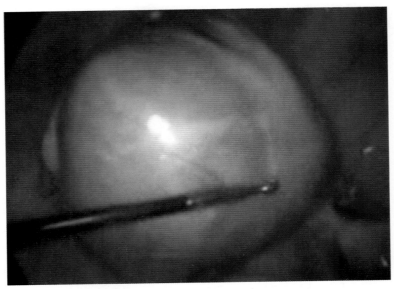

FIGURE 4.17: Fibroid uterus bigger size

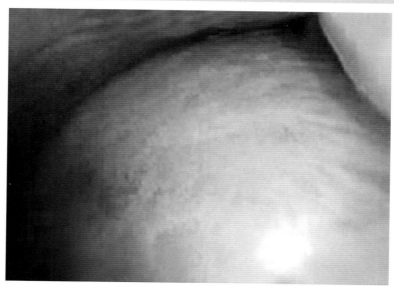

Figure 4.18: 26-28 weeks size uterus

From left lower port insert bipolar and from middle port scissors.

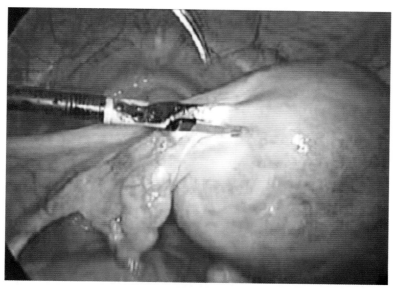

Figure 4.19: Left Site fallopian tube coagulation

I Start from left cornual site. Fallopian tube, ovarian ligament, round ligament and lastly ovarian vessels. About 1-1.5 cm away from cornual so, bleeding becomes less.

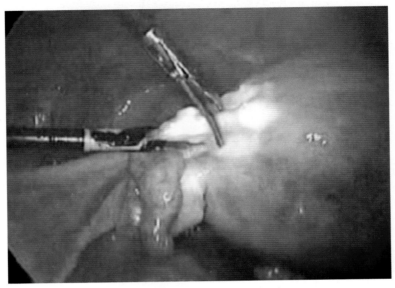

FIGURE 4.20: Cutting of fallopian tube

- Cutting of tube little bit more so, does not come in field (1/3 salpingectomy)
- Fallopian tube, round ligament, ovarian ligament then ovarian vessels complex coagulation and cut.

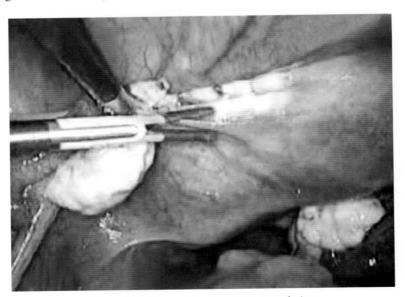

FIGURE 4.21: The ovarian ligament coagulation

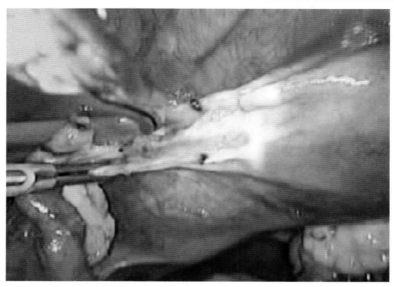

FIGURE 4.22: Cutting of ovarian ligament

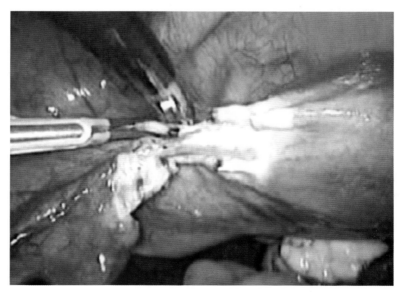

FIGURE 4.23: Round ligament coagulation and cutting

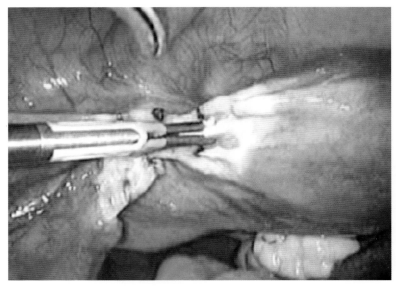

FIGURE 4.24: Ovarian vessels coagulation and cutting. So, bleeding become less

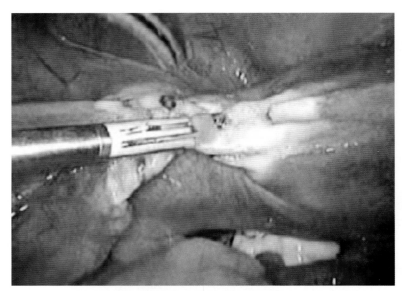

FIGURE 4.25: Coagulation of ascending branch of uterine

- Proper coagulation at cornual angle to prevent back flow bleeding
- I always prefer to remove tubes and ovary latter.

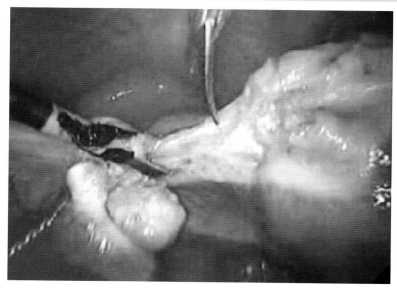

FIGURE 4.26: Then enter in broad ligament

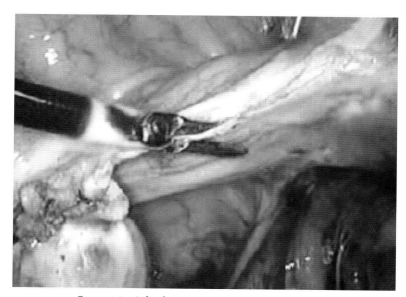

FIGURE 4.27: Lift of posterior layer of broad ligament

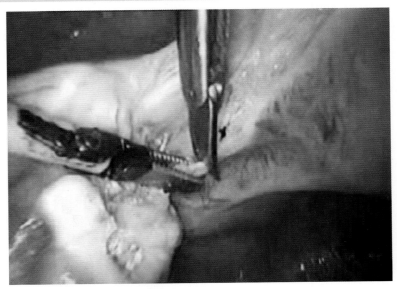

FIGURE 4.28: Opening of posterior layer

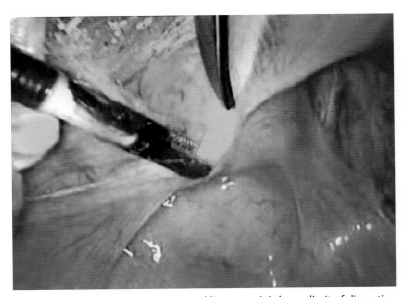

FIGURE 4.29: Dissection upto uterosacral ligament, it is lower limit of dissection

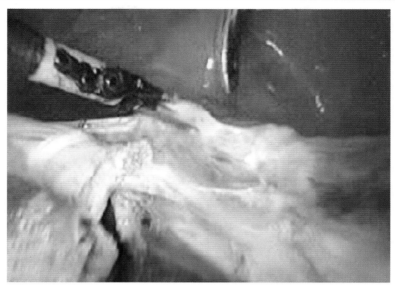

FIGURE 4.30A: Anterior leaf dissection

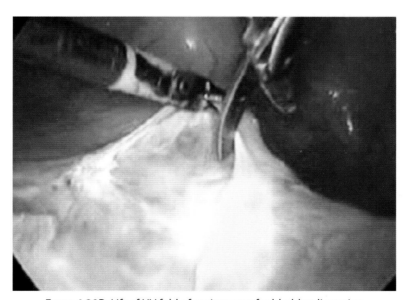

FIGURE 4.30B: Lift of UV fold of peritoneum for bladder dissection

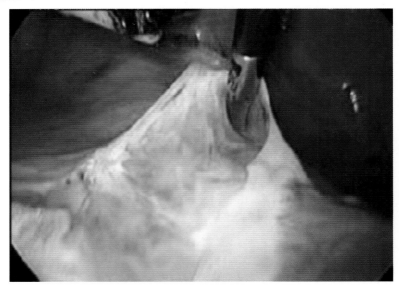

FIGURE 4.31: Dissection of bladder pillars

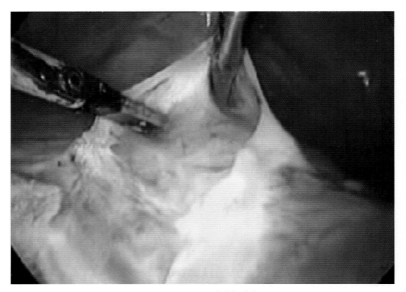

FIGURE 4.32: Push bladder

- Push bladder with help of bipolar and scissor
- No extra steps required for bladder dissection.

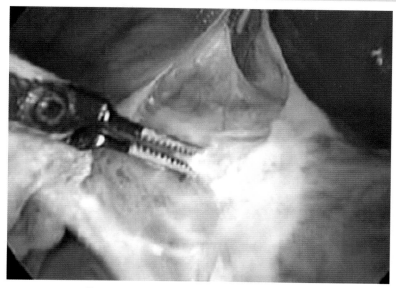

FIGURE 4.33: Skeletonization of uterine vessels

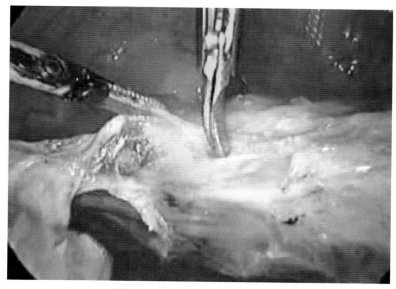

FIGURE 4.34: Uterine vessels seen

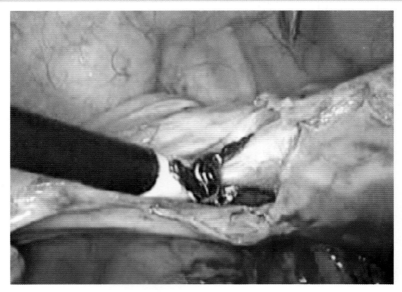

FIGURE **4.35:** Distal coagulation

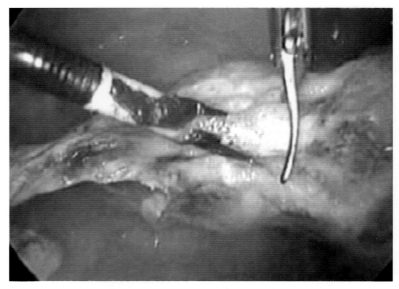

FIGURE **4.36:** Proximal coagulation of vessels

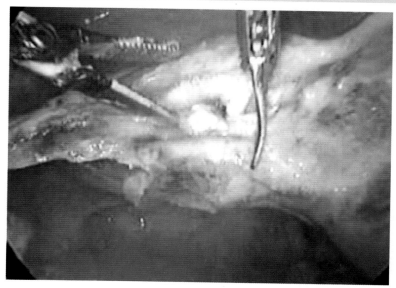

FIGURE **4.37:** Cutting of vessels

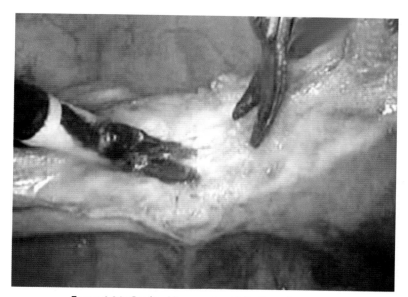

FIGURE **4.38:** Cardinal ligament middle fiber dissection

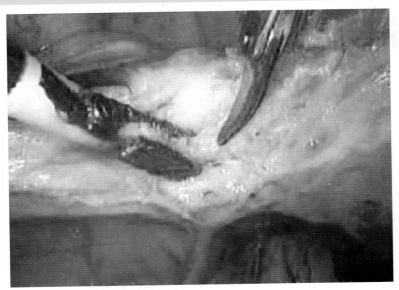

FIGURE 4.39: Cardinal ligament lower fiber dissection

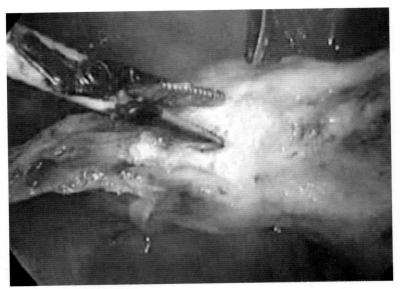

FIGURE 4.40: Cardinal ligament dissection upper fiber dissection

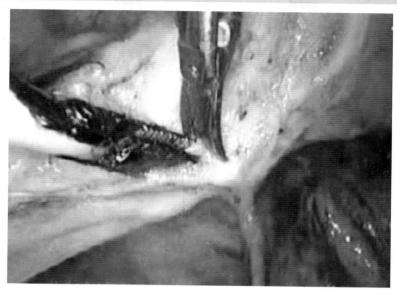

FIGURE **4.41:** Uterosacral dissection

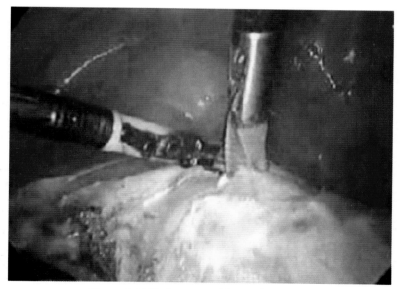

FIGURE **4.42:** Vasicocervcval fascia dissection

- Therefore, one side dissection over
- It completes dissection from left cornual structure, broad ligament, bladder, uterine vessels, cardinal ligament and uterosacral ligament.

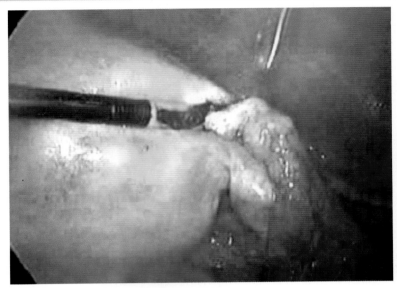

FIGURE 4.43: Right fallopian tube

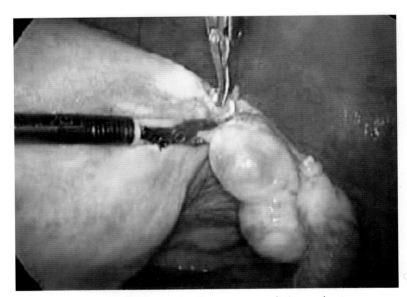

FIGURE 4.44: Right ovarian ligament coagulation and cut

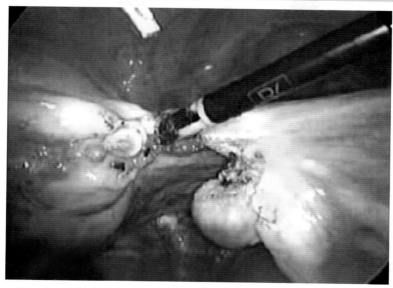

FIGURE 4.45: Coagulation of right ligament

- Right round ligament
- Change of only bipolar forceps.

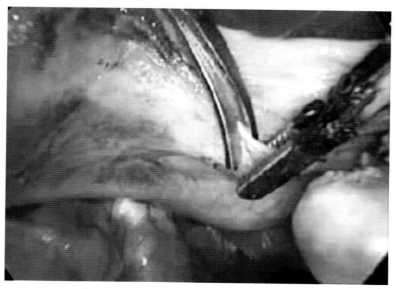

FIGURE 4.46: Posterior layer of broad ligament

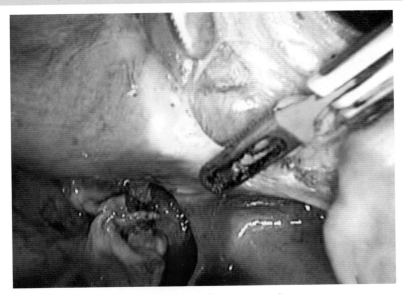

FIGURE 4.47: Dissection of posterior peritoneum

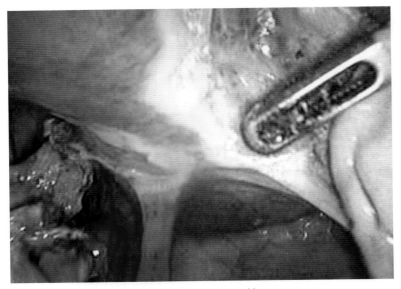

FIGURE 4.48: Right uterosacral ligament

- Lower, limit of dissection on both side seen very nicely
- At the insertion of uterosacral.

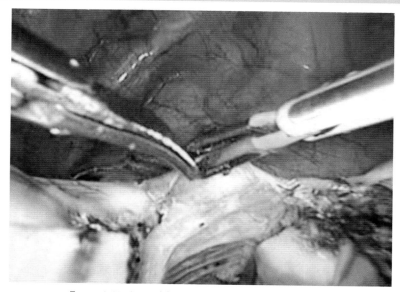

FIGURE **4.49:** Again lift of peritoneum and coagulation

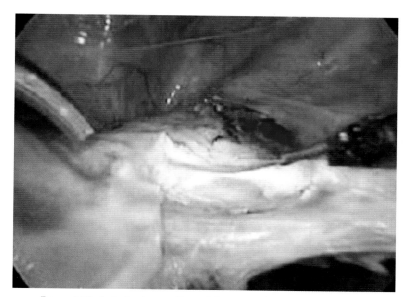

FIGURE **4.50:** Anterior layer of broad ligament dissection completed

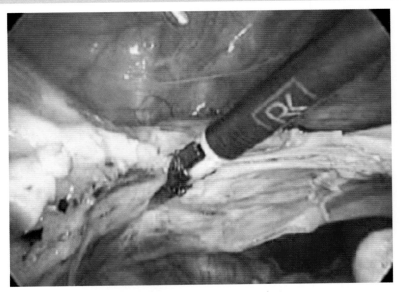

FIGURE **4.51:** Right Uterine coagulation

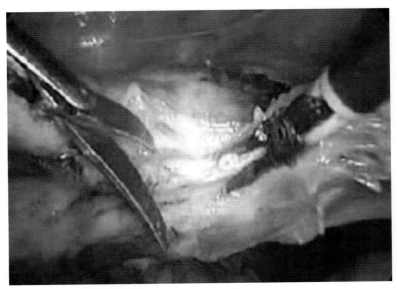

FIGURE **4.52:** Cutting of uterine

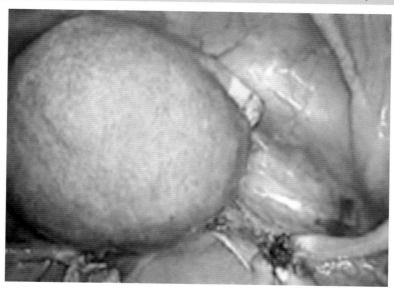

FIGURE 4.53: Pallor uterus after both uterine dissections

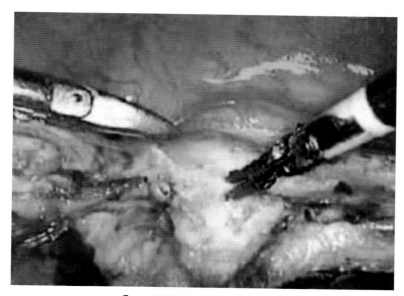

FIGURE 4.54: Ligament dissection

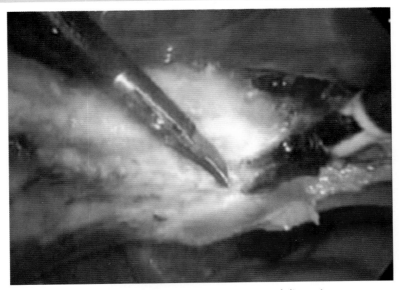

FIGURE **4.55:** Cardinal ligament + Uterosacral dissection

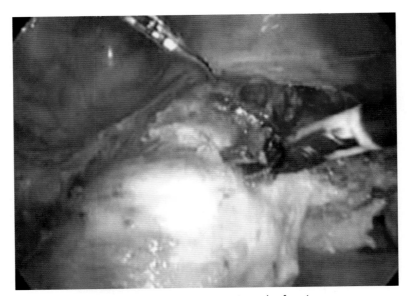

FIGURE **4.56:** Only remain part is vault of vagina

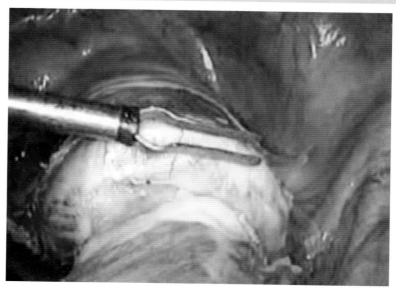

FIGURE 4.57: Coagulation of vaginal margin

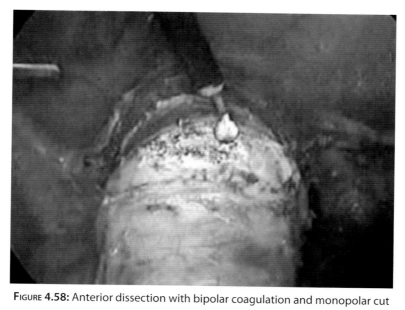

FIGURE 4.58: Anterior dissection with bipolar coagulation and monopolar cut

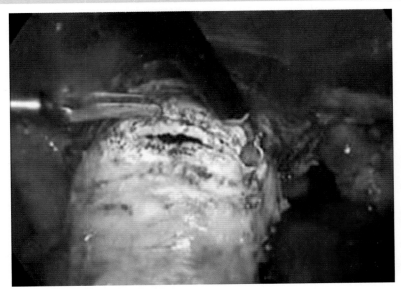

FIGURE **4.59:** Lateral coagulation and cut

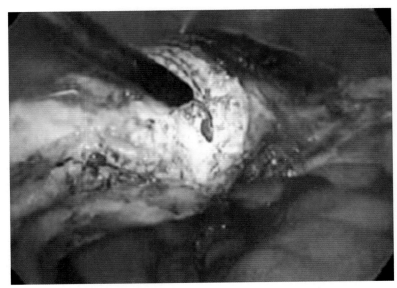

FIGURE **4.60:** Right lateral

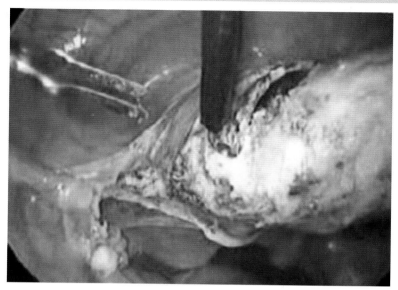

FIGURE 4.61: Left lateral dissection

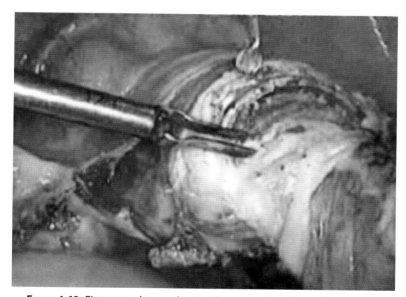

FIGURE 4.62: First coagulate and cut with monopolar electrode or scissor

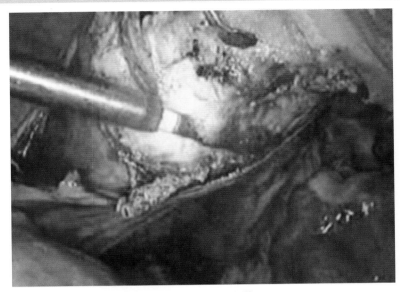

FIGURE **4.63:** Coagulation of ligament

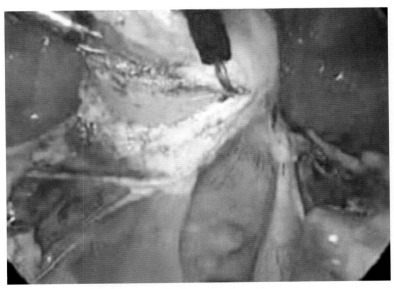

FIGURE **4.64:** Posterior dissection

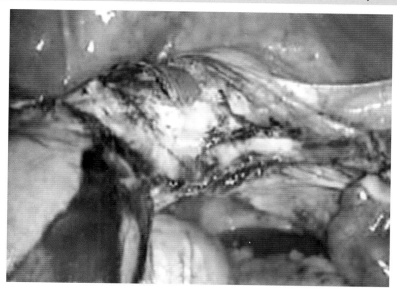

FIGURE **4.65:** Now proceed for right side dissection

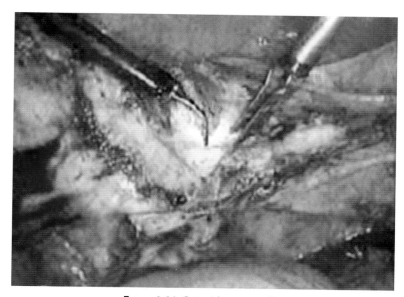

FIGURE **4.66:** Cut with monopolar

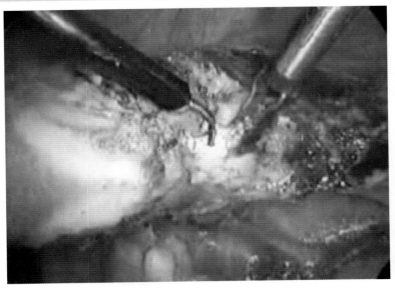

FIGURE 4.67: Last part of dissection

- Change of only bipolar forceps
- Last dissection.

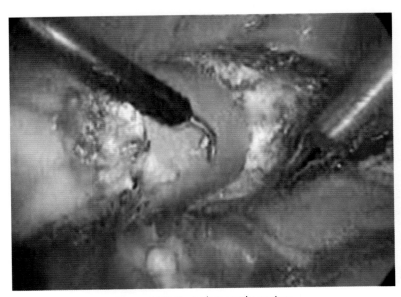

FIGURE 4.68: Complete vault cutting

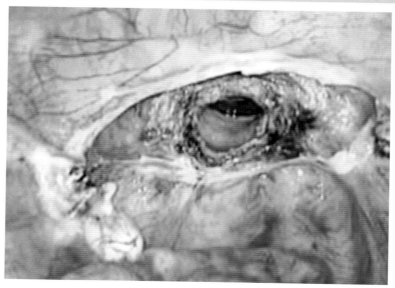

FIGURE **4.69**: Complete TLH

- See bloodless view
- Maintaining of pericervical ring for support.

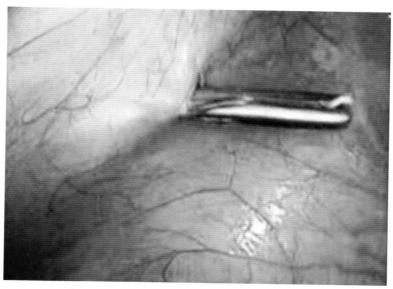

FIGURE **4.70**: Insertion of suture inside the abdomen

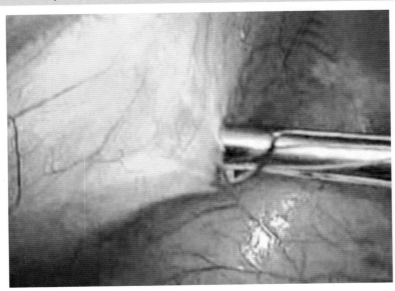

FIGURE 4.71: Harry- rich technique of suture needle insertion

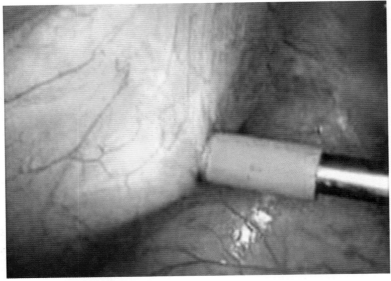

FIGURE 4.72: First suture insertion with needle then sleeves insertion

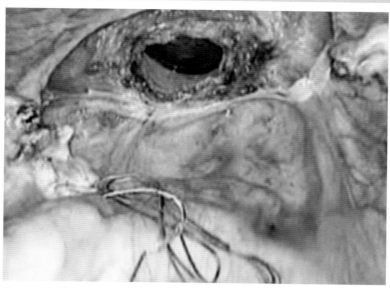

FIGURE 4.73: Insertion of suture as it is from foil. So, make it very easy handling

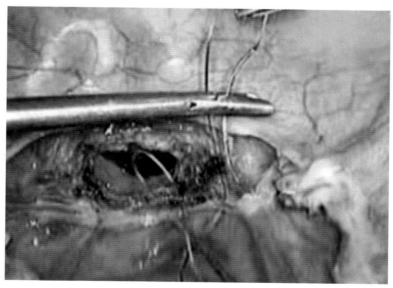

FIGURE 4.74: Needle hold at right angle

- Contralateral suturing. One needle holder and other tooth serrated grasper
- Hold needle at anterior 2/3rd and posterior 1/3rd.

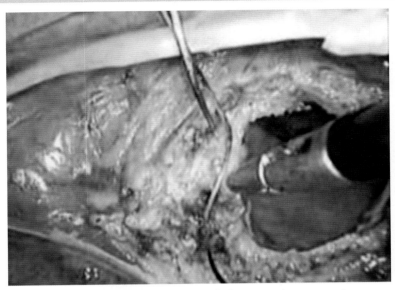

FIGURE 4.75: At left angle, pass needle from anterior to posterior

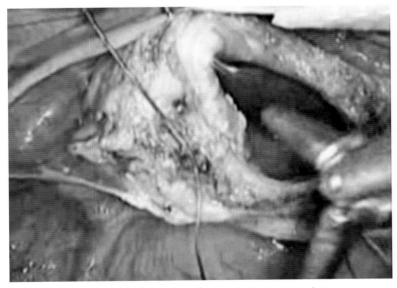

FIGURE 4.76: Needle pass from anterior to posterior

- Grasper is helpful in holding tissue
- And take adequate bite.

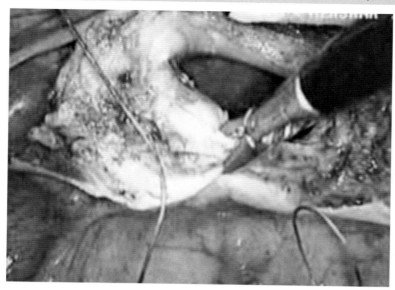

FIGURE 4.77: Posterior

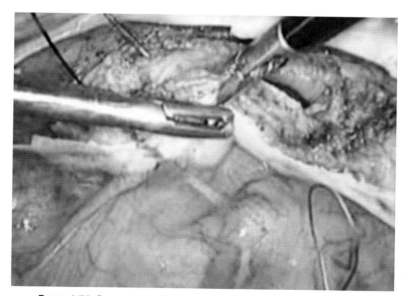

FIGURE 4.78: Remove needle in curve fashion so, less tissue damage

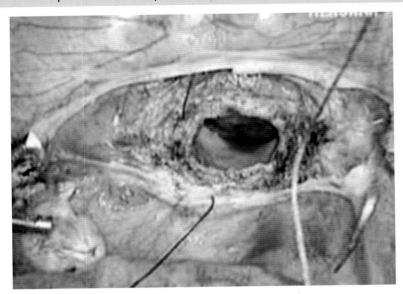

FIGURE **4.79:** Thread pulls on opposite side

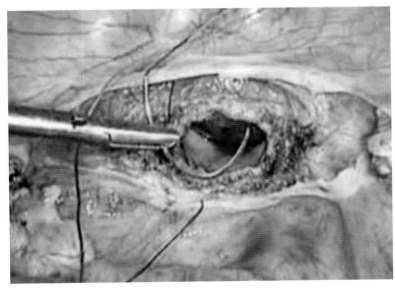

FIGURE **4.80:** Again, pass needle in same way

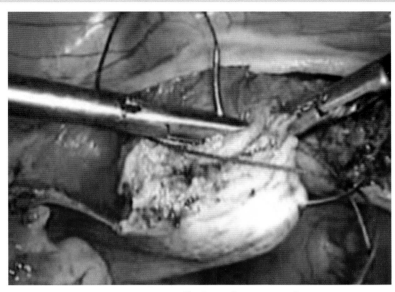

FIGURE 4.81: Needle through uterosacral

- Taking Uterosacral
- Help in vault suspension.

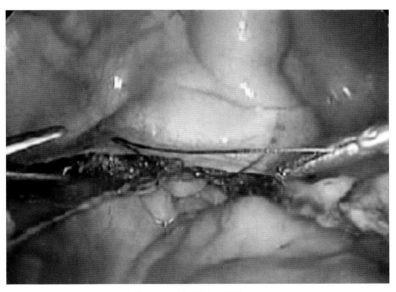

FIGURE 4.82: Make "C" loop

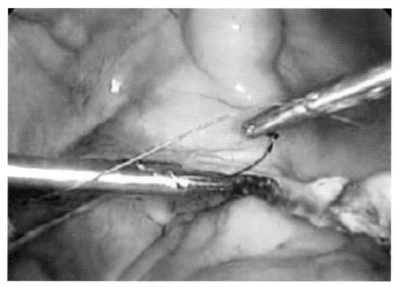

FIGURE **4.83:** Up and down movements

- Up down movement of needle holder and grasper
- Needle holder down and grasper up.

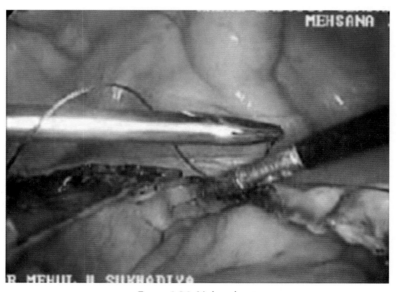

FIGURE **4.84:** Make a loop

- Needle holder up and grasper down
- Help in formation of wind.

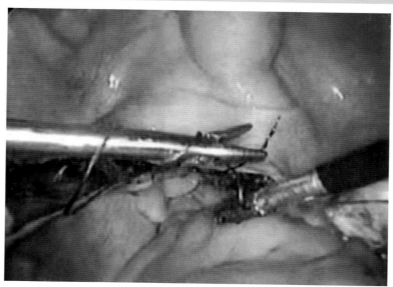

FIGURE **4.85:** Grasp shorter end

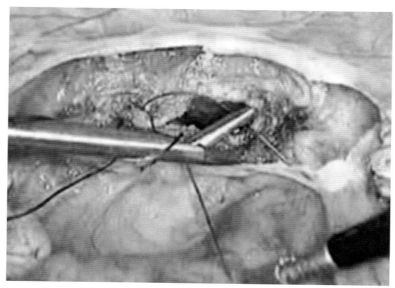

FIGURE **4.86:** Two-thirds around needle holder

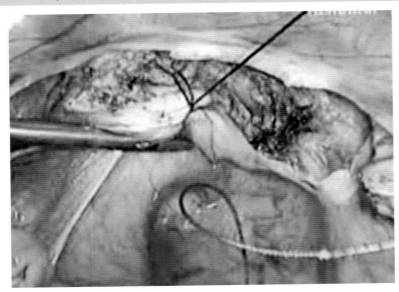

FIGURE **4.87:** Tie note

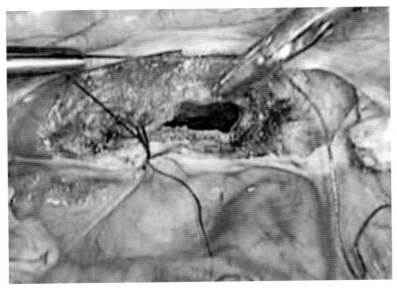

FIGURE **4.88:** Again, make loop "C" or "U"

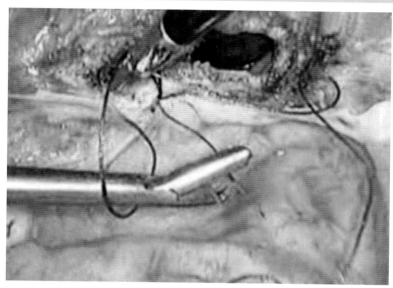

FIGURE **4.89:** One-third half hitch

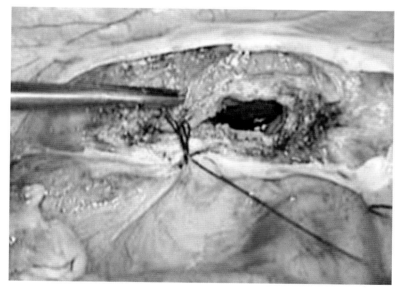

FIGURE **4.90:** Tie

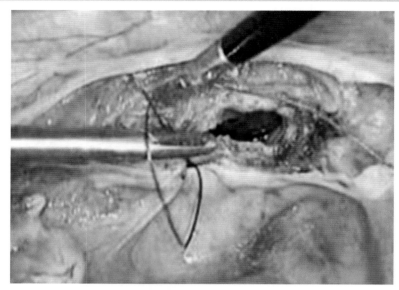

FIGURE **4.91:** Again one-third half hitch in reverse direction

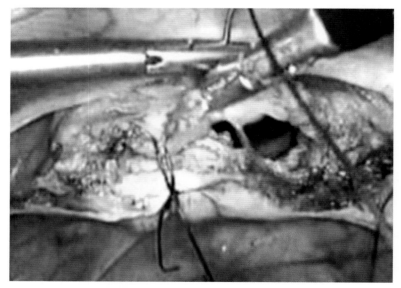

FIGURE **4.92:** So, final surgeon note complete

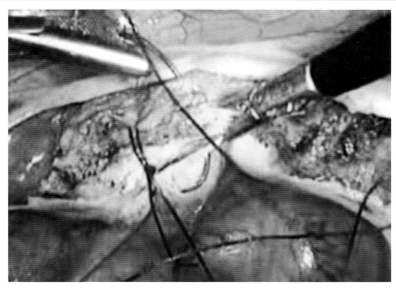

FIGURE **4.93:** After that taking of one-third of vault part

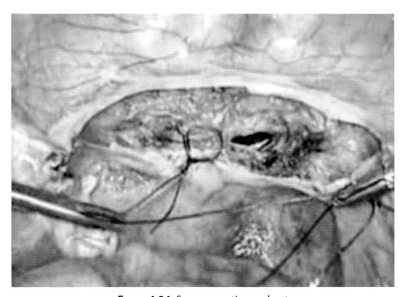

FIGURE **4.94:** Same way, ties and cut

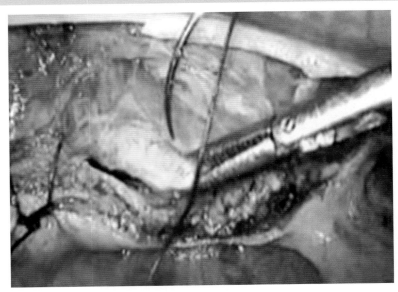

FIGURE **4.95:** Right angle suturing

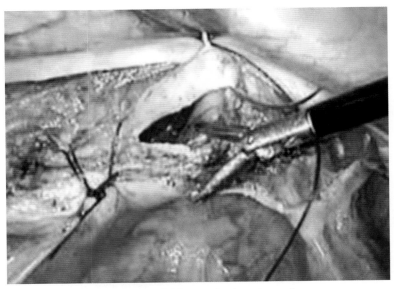

FIGURE **4.96:** Taking angle–Anterior wall

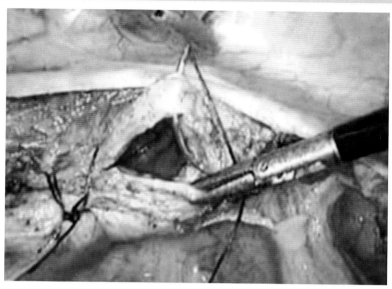

FIGURE 4.97: Posterior wall

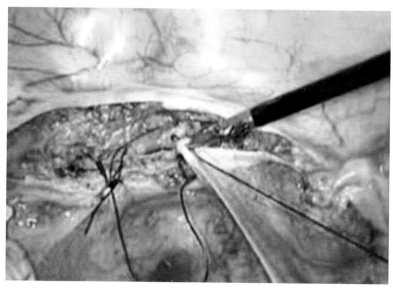

FIGURE 4.98: Taking uterosacral

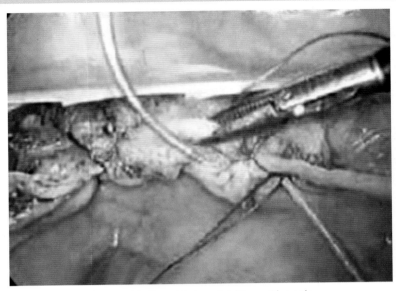

FIGURE **4.99:** One-third vault taking with angle

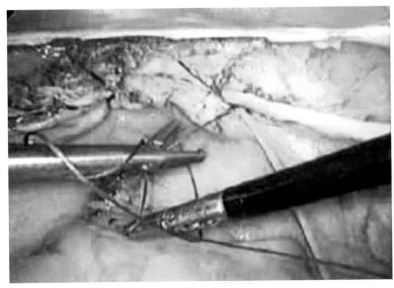

FIGURE **4.100:** Final stitch

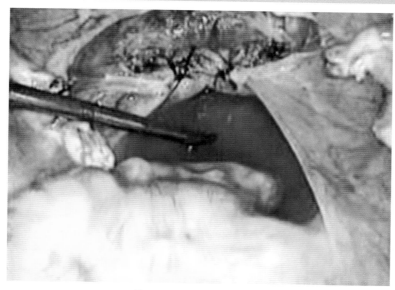

FIGURE 4.101: Saline wash

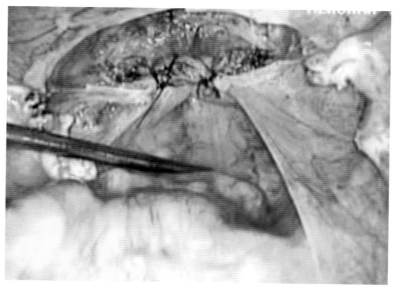

FIGURE 4.102: Clear lavage

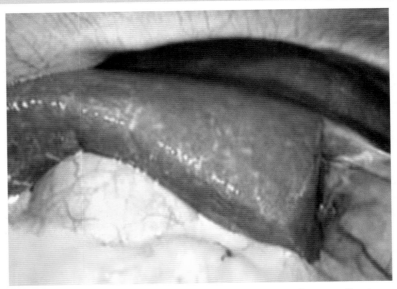

FIGURE **4.103:** Always-liver bad examination after surgery for any collection

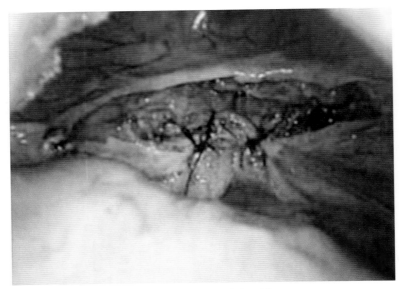

FIGURE **4.104:** Examination of pedicle without pneumo

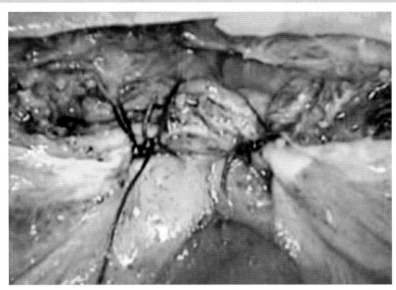

FIGURE **4.105:** Post hysterectomy clear fluid .not a single drop of blood seen

CHAPTER
5
Difficult Total Laparoscopic Hysterectomy

A. TOTAL LAPAROSCOPIC HYSTERECTOMY WITH PREVIOUS LOWER SEGMENT CESARIAN SECTION

Case-1

- Whenever we deal with previous section TLH, we always fear of bladder. Therefore, careful dissection of bladder is must. Bladder adhesion of scar site depends on technique of CS, healing tendency and any segmental complication at the time of CS.

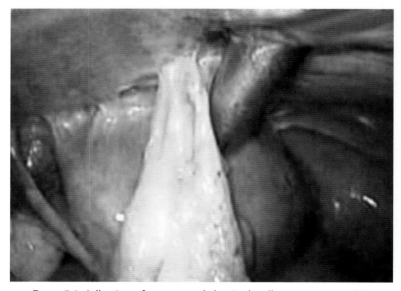

FIGURE 5.1: Adhesion of uterus on abdominal wall—preoperative LSCS

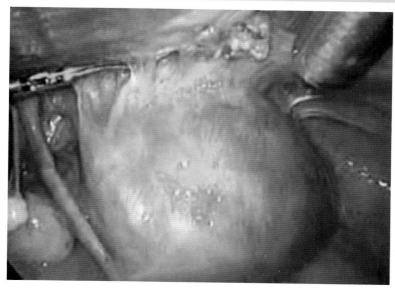

FIGURE 5.2: Separation of omentum band

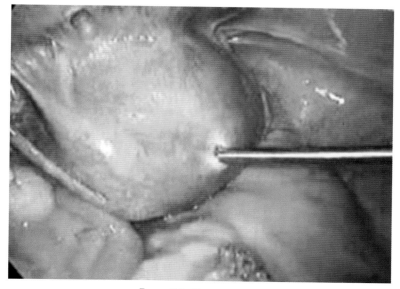

FIGURE 5.3: Myomo screw

- Myoma screw fixation for manipulation.
- In this case uterus densely adherent to anterior abdominal wall.
- So vaginal manipulation not possible.
- Cervix higher up.

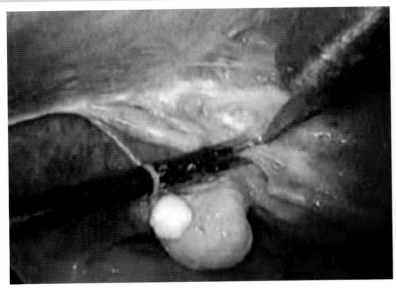

FIGURE 5.4: Start with cornual dissection

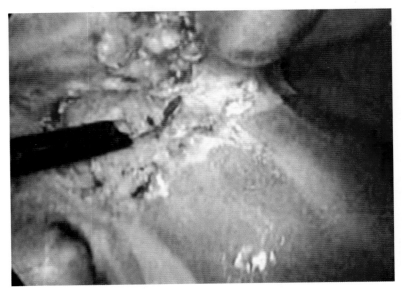

FIGURE 5.5: Dissection of adhesion

- Dissection with monopolar.
- Try to make normal anatomy.

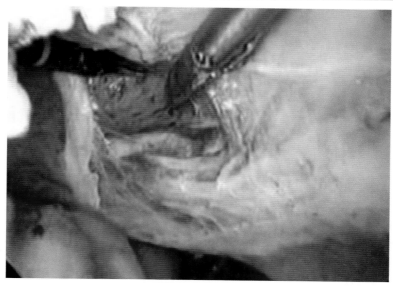

FIGURE 5.6: Anterior to uterine

- Enter in lateral space for bladder dissection
- For lateral space dissection just go above uterine.

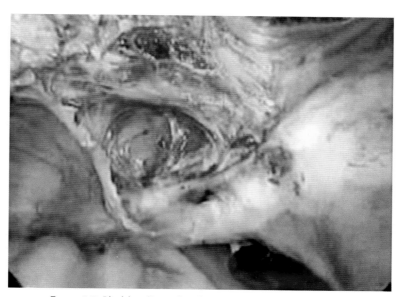

FIGURE 5.7: Bladder distend with saline for border assessment

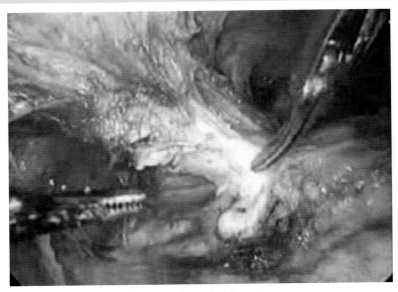

FIGURE 5.8: Stepwise dissection

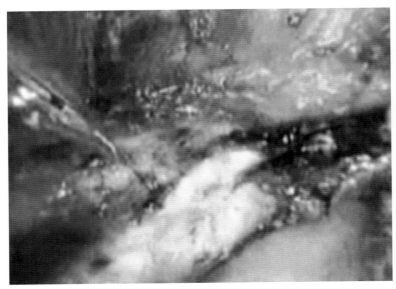

FIGURE 5.9: Bladder completely dissected out

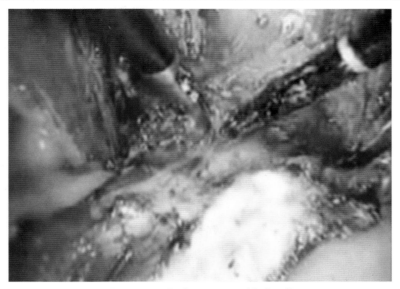

FIGURE 5.10: Both uterine tackled well

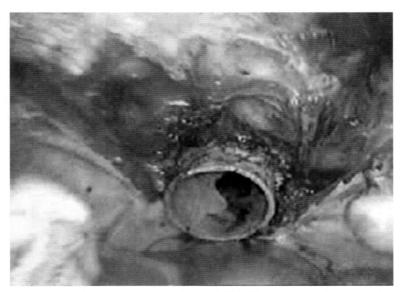

FIGURE 5.11: Complete TLH in such cases we have to do careful bladder dissection because it is adherent to uterus

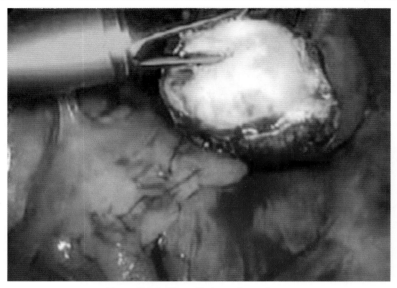

Figure 5.12: Morcellation of specimen

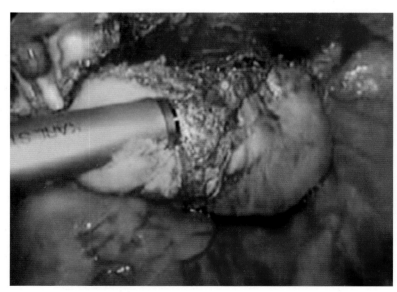

Figure 5.13: Morcellation

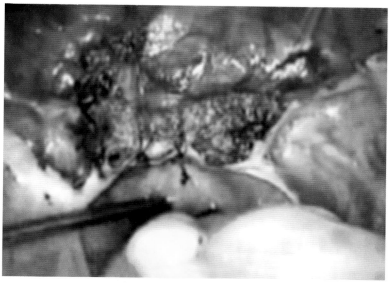

FIGURE 5.14: Hysterectomy over

Case-2

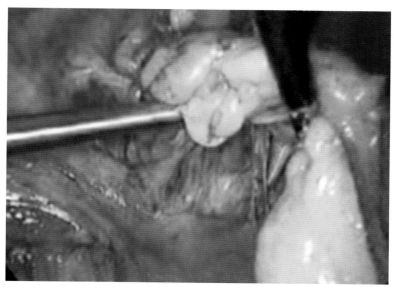

FIGURE 5.15: Omentum adherent to CS scar

- Omentum adherent at UV fold with previous CS scar
- Do adhesiolysis and go for hysterectomy

Separation of bladder in different ways:
1. Lateral dissection–bipolar and scissors
2. Middle dissection
3. Sharp dissection with scissors and suction
4. With harmonic
5. Monopolar.

Case-3

I always prefer lateral dissection and SOS sharp dissection.

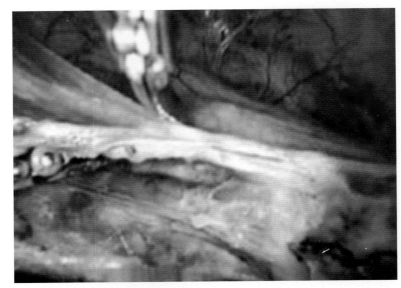

FIGURE 5.16: Left uterine vessels and bladder adhesion

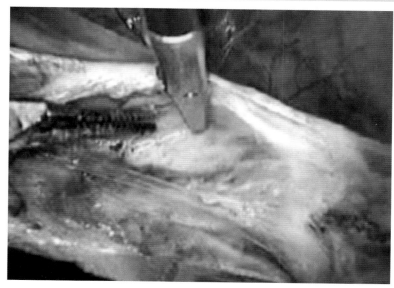

FIGURE **5.17:** Entry point–just above uterine vessels

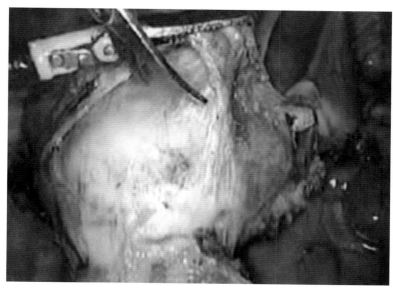

FIGURE **5.18:** Cutting of bladder pillars

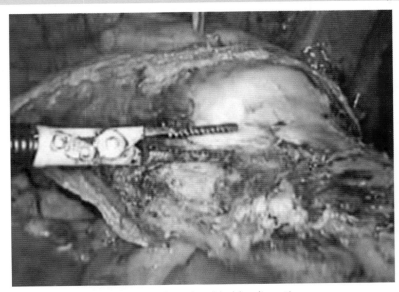

FIGURE 5.19: Complete bladder dissection

Case-4

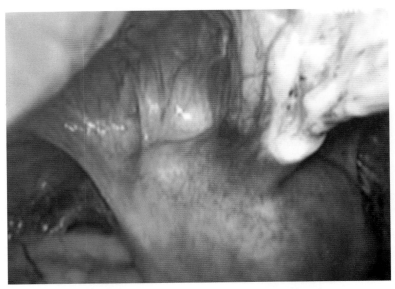

FIGURE 5.20: Uterus with anterior abdominal band

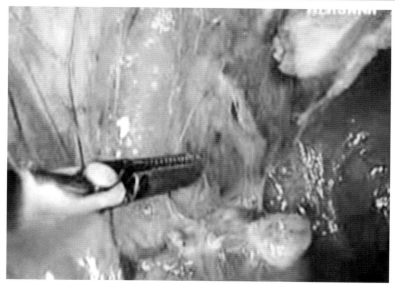

Figure 5.21: Cutting of bands and bladder dissection

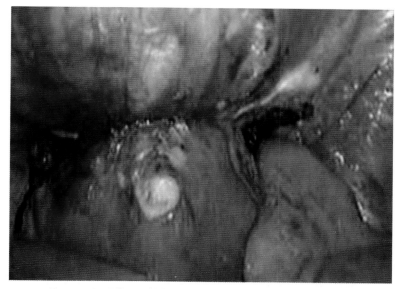

Figure 5.22: Filling of bladder with saline for level assessment

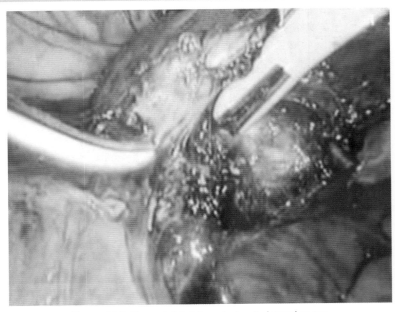

FIGURE 5.23: From right side entering in lateral space

Case-5

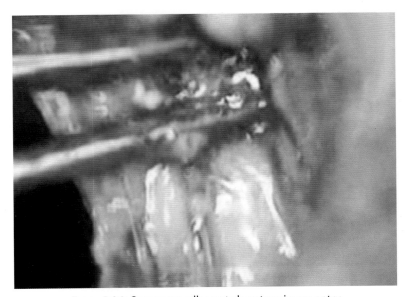

FIGURE 5.24: Omentum adherent close to primary entry

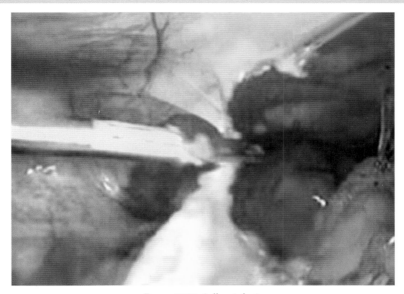

FIGURE 5.25: Adhesiolysis

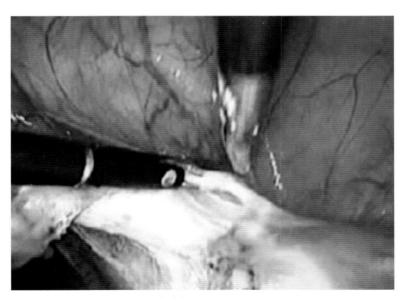

FIGURE 5.26: Bladder peritoneum separation

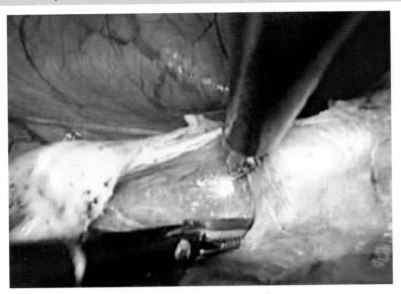

FIGURE 5.27: Good avascular lateral space

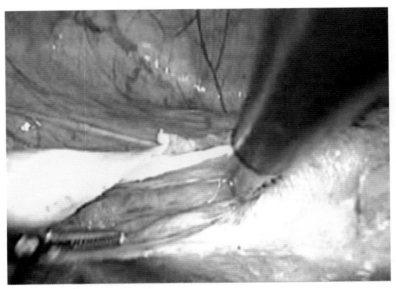

FIGURE 5.28: Uterine seen

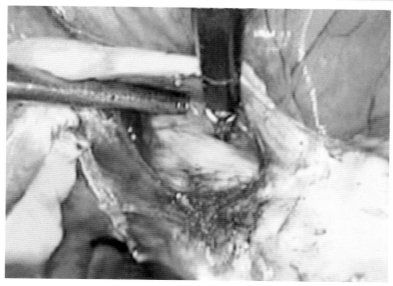

FIGURE 5.29: Bladder completely separated from cervix

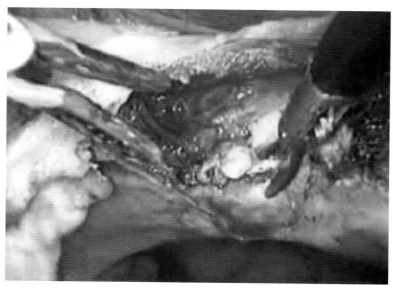

FIGURE 5.30: Then left uterine coagulated and cut

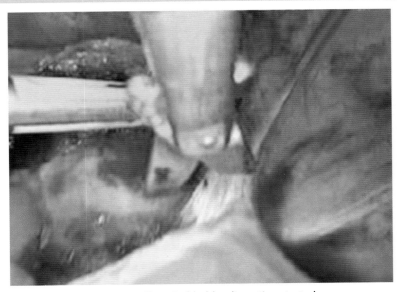

FIGURE 5.31: Remain bladder dissection started

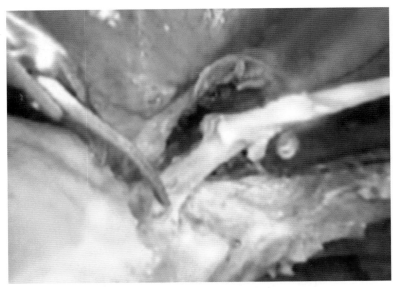

FIGURE 5.32: Right side dissection of bladder

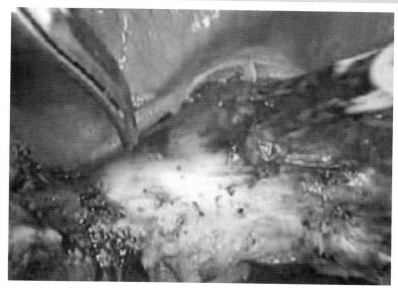

FIGURE 5.33: The bladder completely separated

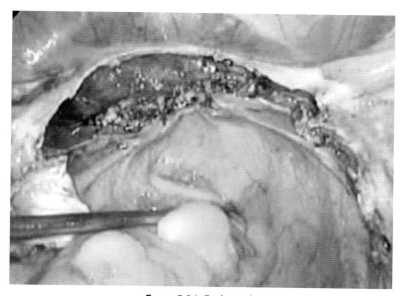

FIGURE 5.34: End result

Cystoscopic Examination After Difficult Bladder Dissection

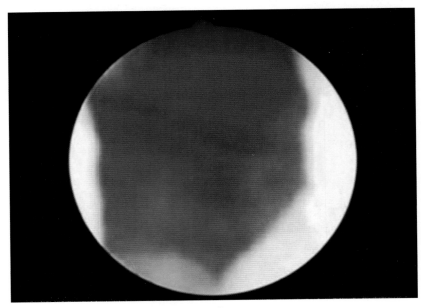

FIGURE 5.35: Cystoscopy

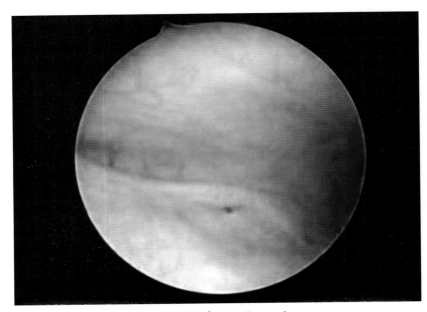

FIGURE 5.36: Left ureteric opening

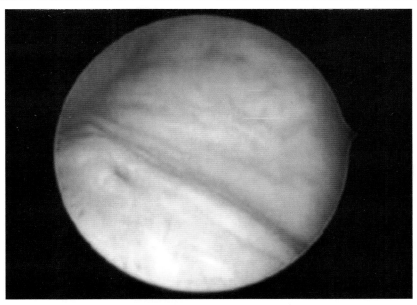

FIGURE 5.37: Right ureteric opening

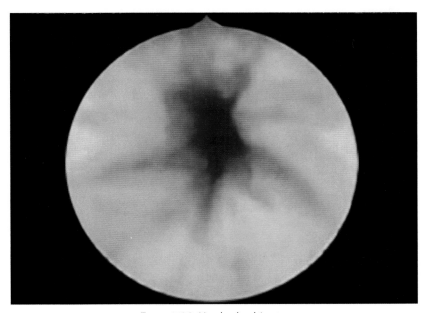

FIGURE 5.38: Urethral sphincter

B. UTERUS WITH BIGGER SIZE

Case-6

- In that circumstances after primary entry, proper assessment of uterus size, position and anteroposterior diameter we have to choose secondary port at higher level.
- Some cases we have to change primary port into secondary port and primary just near xephoid process under vision.
- Then proceed in same way.

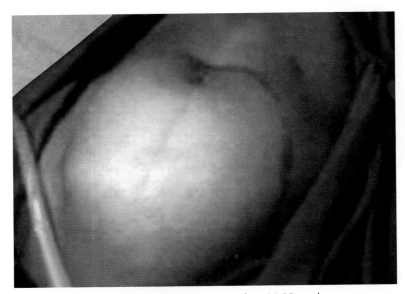

FIGURE 5.39: Size of uterus more than 26-28 weeks

FIGURE 5.40: Could not see any space to work

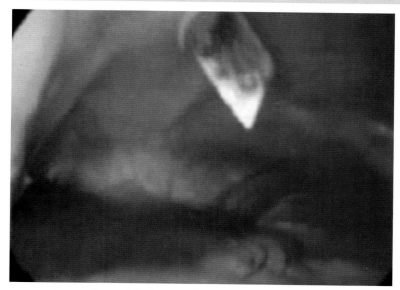

FIGURE 5.41: Port just below xephoid process

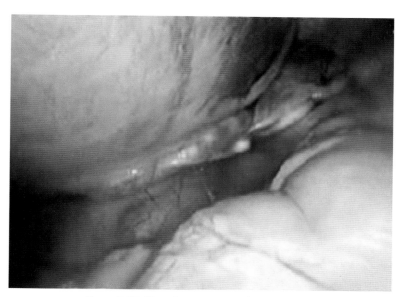

FIGURE 5.42: Size of uterus more than 26 weeks

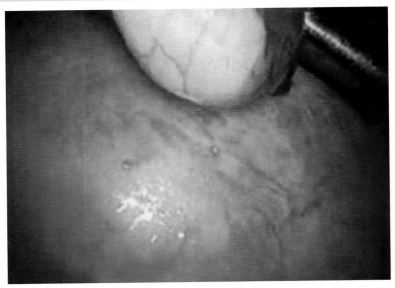

FIGURE 5.43: Primary port seen

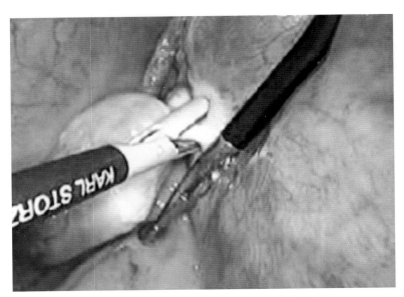

FIGURE 5.44: Ovarian ligament-coagulation

- All ports are at higher level
- Due to bigger size all ligaments much distorted in anatomy and pedicle become large and thick, so need of proper coagulation to prevent bleeding.

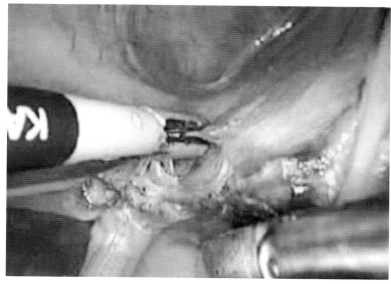

FIGURE 5.45: Anterior leaf of broad ligament

- IP Ligament coagulated and cut
- Enter in broad ligament leaves.

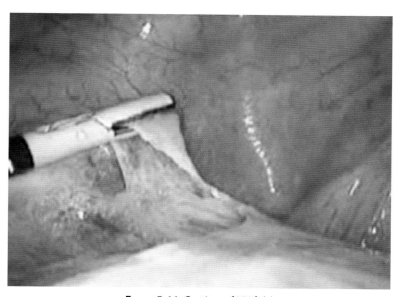

FIGURE 5.46: Cutting of UV fold

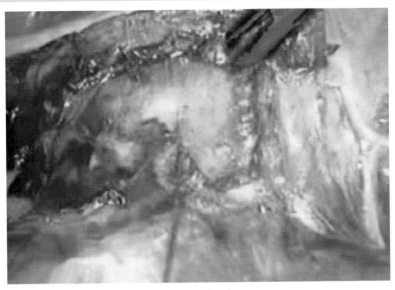

FIGURE **5.47:** Bladder dissection

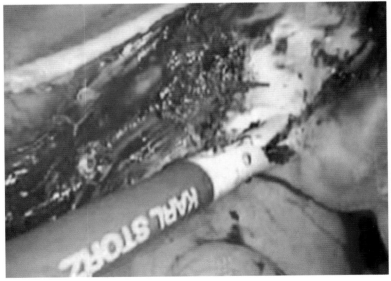

FIGURE **5.48:** Left uterine cutting

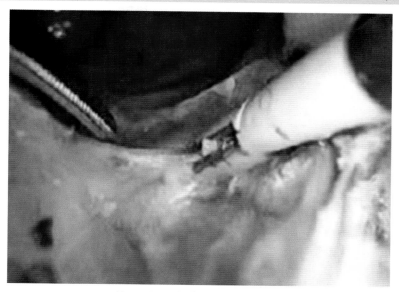

FIGURE 5.49: Right side dissection

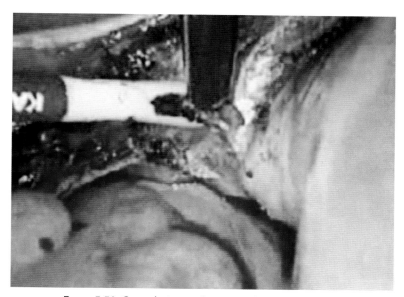

FIGURE 5.50: Coagulation and cutting of vault on left side

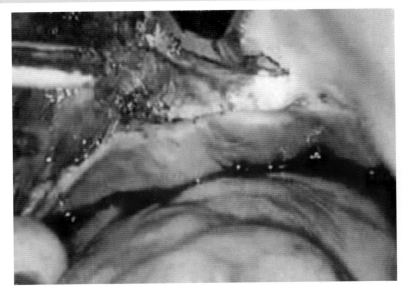

Figure 5.51: Posterior dissection

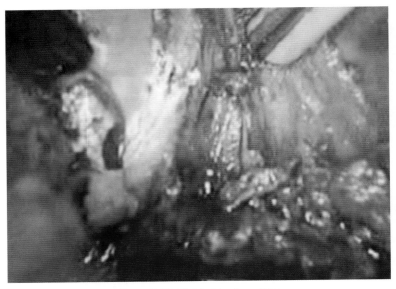

Figure 5.52: Right side dissection

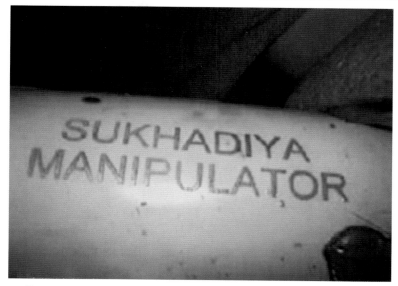

FIGURE 5.53: Our manipulator helpful in manipulating any size of uterus

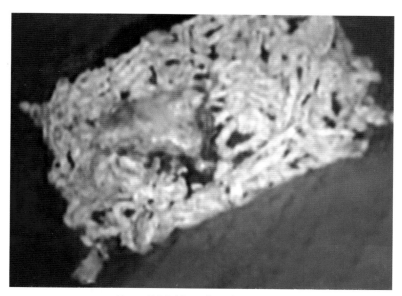

FIGURE 5.54: Morcellated specimen

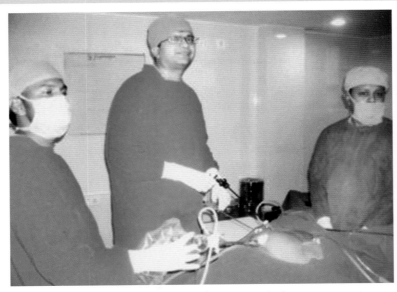

FIGURE 5.55: RADHE endoscopy surgical team

C. PATIENT HAVING SEVERE ENDOMETRIOSIS

- First, do adhesiolysis and then start TLH
- But in some cases, we cannot able to perform adhesiolysis in that case do
- Dissections flush to the uterus and prevent injuries to near vital structures
- Chances of injuries more with this type of case, because inflammatory reaction
- Lead to puckering of surrounding structure
- So, ureter-rectum-Pouch of Douglas-uterus-tubes and ovary everything stuck up.

Case-7

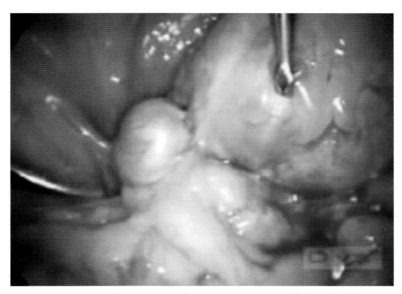

Figure 5.56: Sigmoid + uterus + tube + ovary + rectum all densely adherent

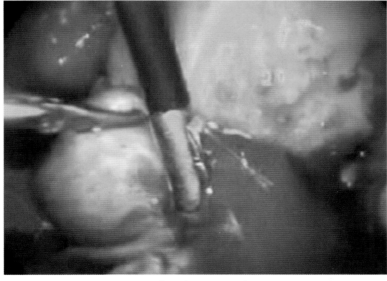

Figure 5.57: Chocolate material came out

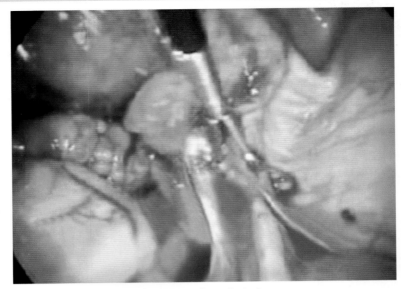

FIGURE 5.58: Adhesiolysis done

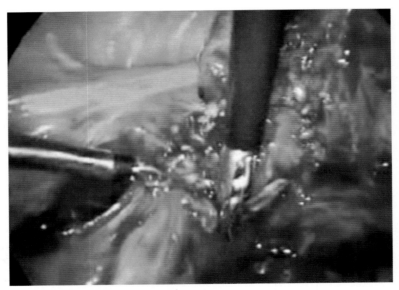

FIGURE 5.59: Then, TLH start

Case-8

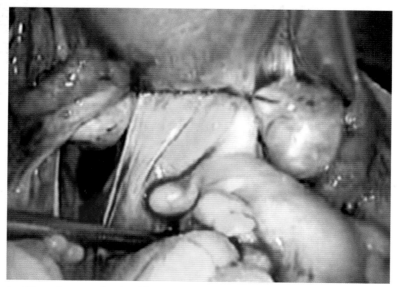

FIGURE 5.60: In this case Pouch of Douglas completely obliterated and rectum, tubes, ovaries, ureteres and uterus are densely adherent

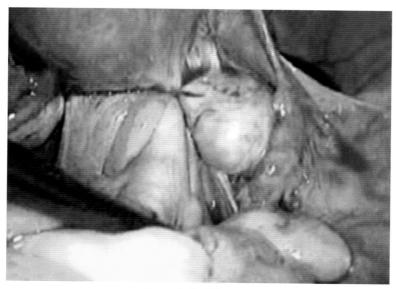

FIGURE 5.61: Adhesion

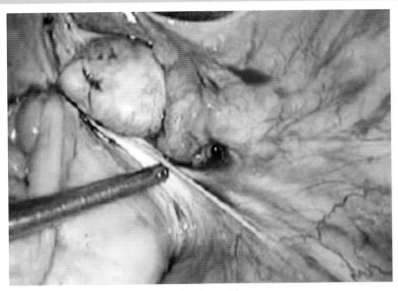

FIGURE **5.62:** Ureter involve

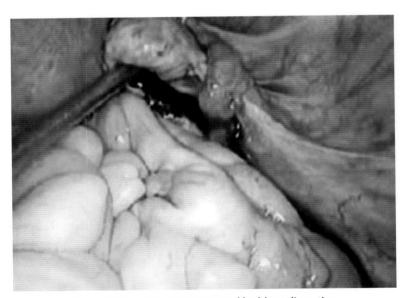

FIGURE **5.63:** Right ovary separated by blunt dissection

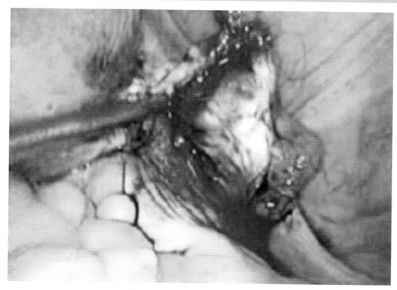

FIGURE **5.64:** Ovary separated

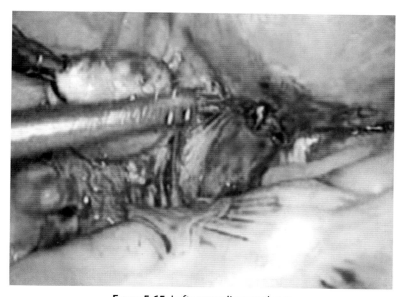

FIGURE **5.65:** Left ovary dissected out

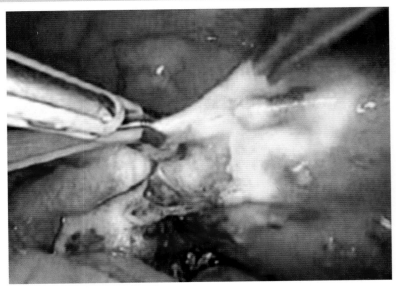

Figure 5.66: After adhesiolysis start TLH

- Then hysterectomy started
- Cornual separation.

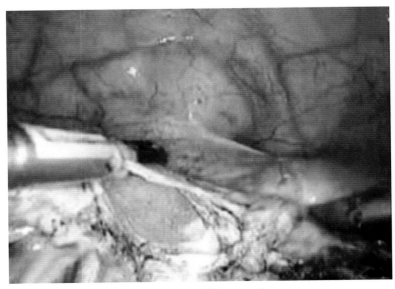

Figure 5.67: UV fold separation

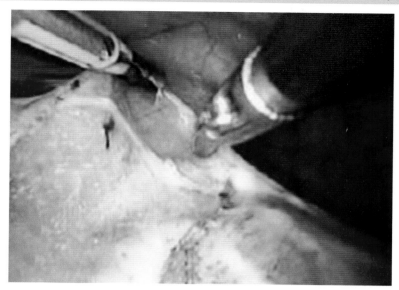

Figure 5.68: Bladder separation

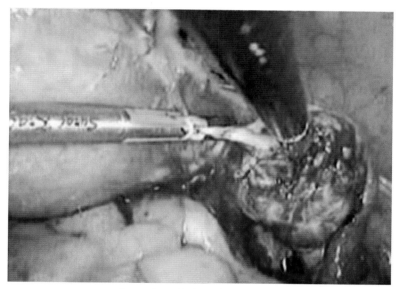

Figure 5.69: Right side dissection

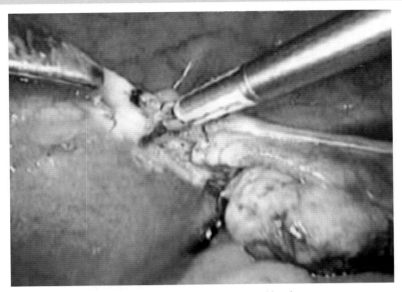

FIGURE 5.70: Cornual structure coagulated by three steps

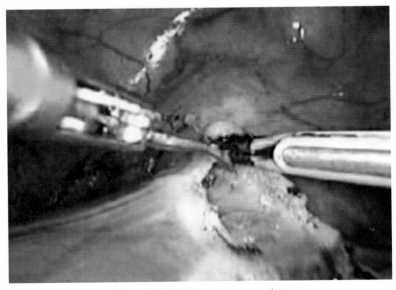

FIGURE 5.71: Peritoneum separation

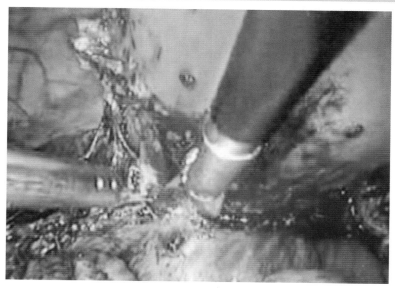

FIGURE 5.72: Sharp dissection to separate rectum

- Separation of rectum by blunt dissection
- Only after both side coagulation of uterine.

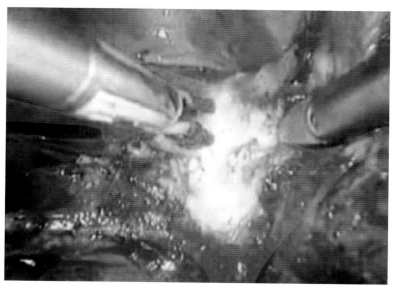

FIGURE 5.73: Cutting of uterine

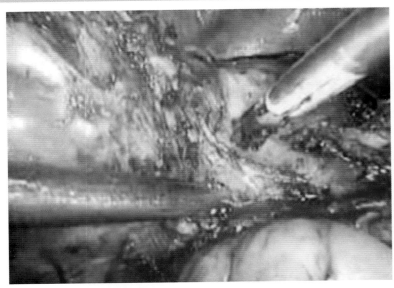

Figure 5.74: Right side uterine and ligament

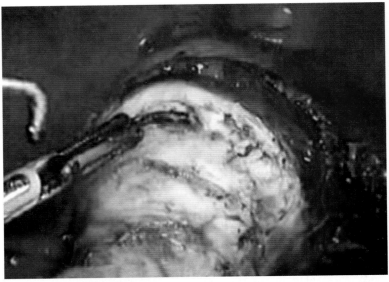

Figure 5.75: Anterior vault cutting

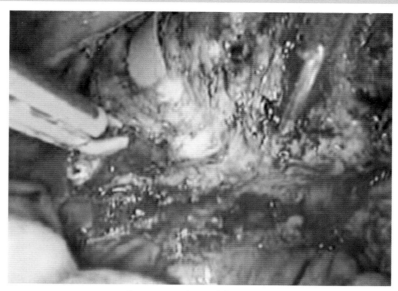

Figure 5.76: Lateral dissection

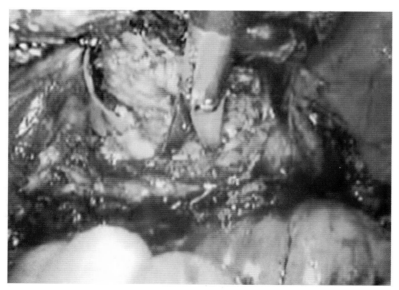

Figure 5.77: Sharp dissection for separation of rectum from vagina

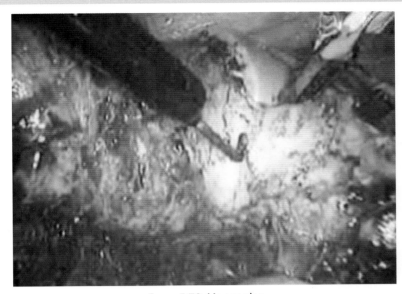

FIGURE 5.78: Monopolar

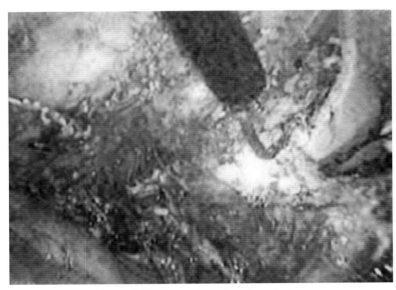

FIGURE 5.79: Separation of vault posterior

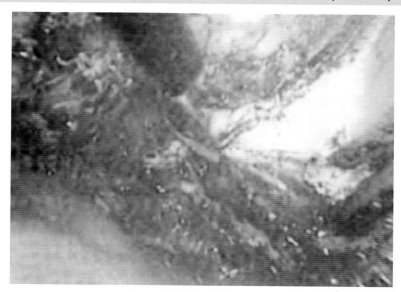

FIGURE 5.80: End of dissection

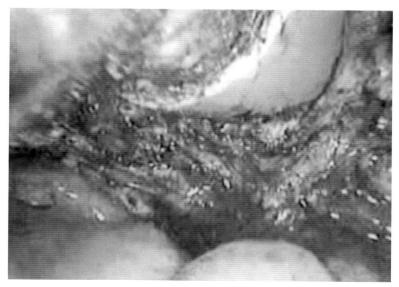

FIGURE 5.81: Complete dissection

- Completed dissection
- Care only requires is proper separation of rectum before using of any energy sources.

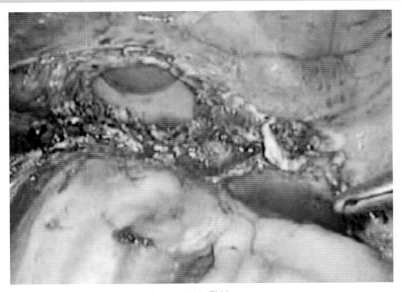

Figure 5.82: TLH over

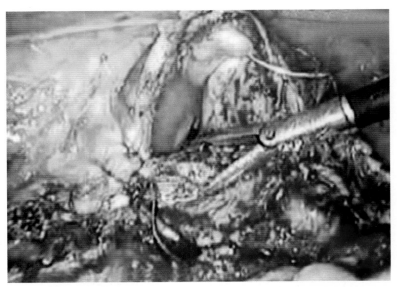

Figure 5.83: Suturing of vault with centicry 1 no 45 cm 40 mm needle

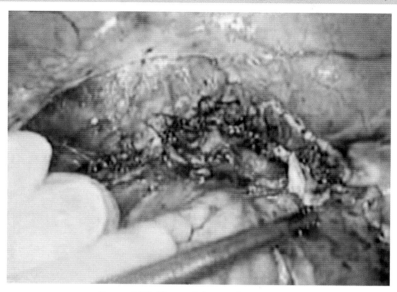

FIGURE **5.84:** Through lavage is necessary

Uterine Prolapse

- Tackle with laparoscopic hysterectomy and economic suspension surgery
- No mash
- No taker fixation.

Case-9

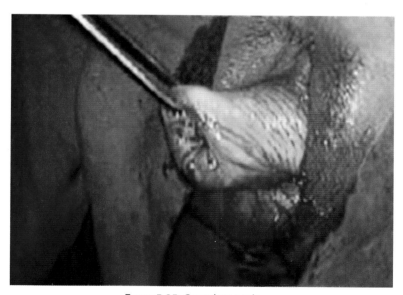

FIGURE **5.85:** Complete prolapse

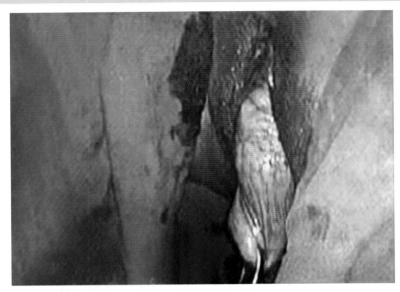

FIGURE 5.86: Cystocele

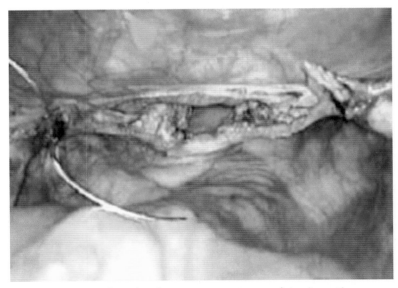

FIGURE 5.87: Complete hysterectomy as we are doing in routine

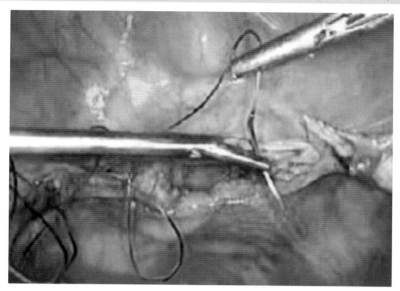

FIGURE 5.88: Vault closer

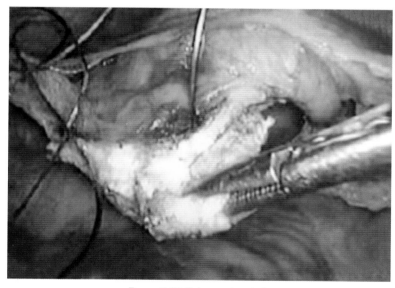

FIGURE 5.89: Take angle stitch

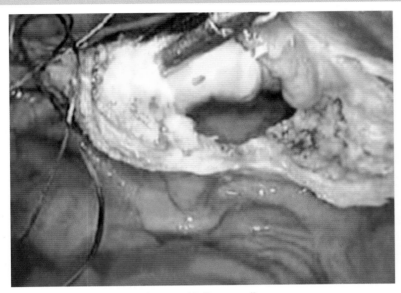

FIGURE 5.90: Pass needle

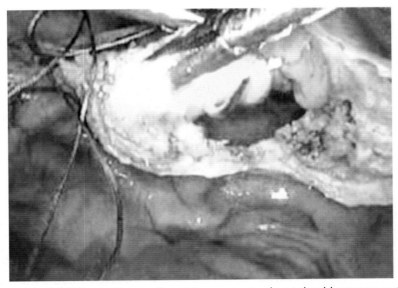

FIGURE 5.91: While passing needle, wrist movement only, no shoulder movement

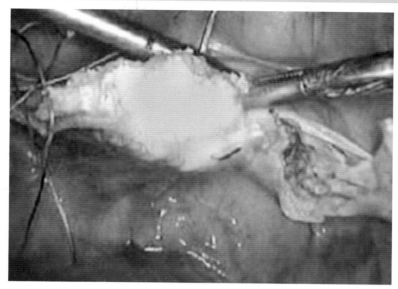

FIGURE 5.92: Taking uterosacral ligament

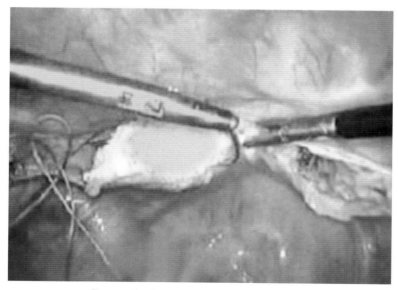

FIGURE 5.93: Remove needle in curve fashion

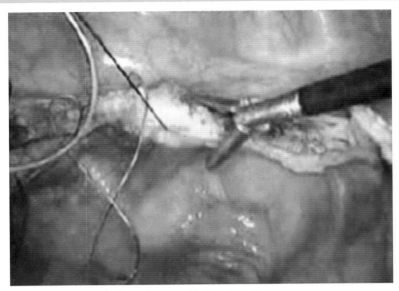

Figure 5.94: Pull thread

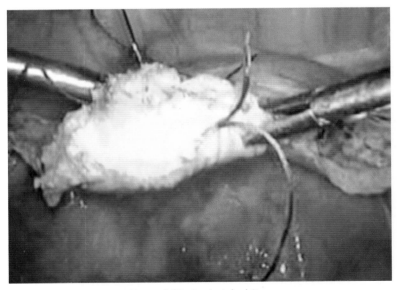

Figure 5.95: Again take bites

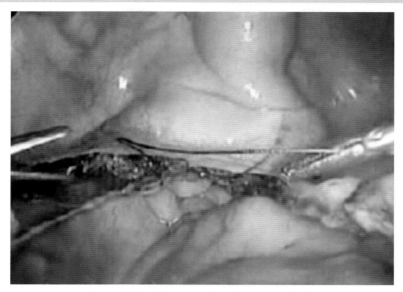

Figure 5.96: C-Loop creation for proper winds

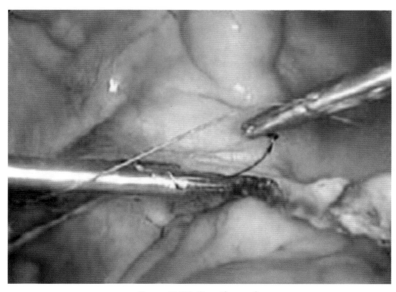

Figure 5.97: One through

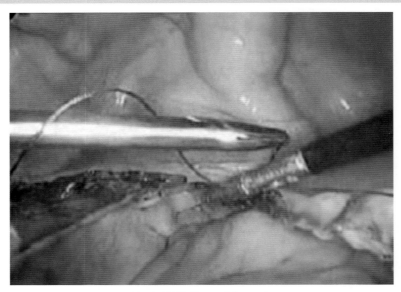

FIGURE 5.98: Second through

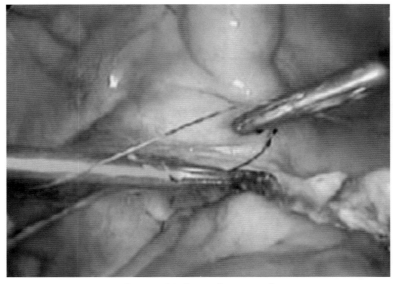

FIGURE 5.99: Grasp shorter end

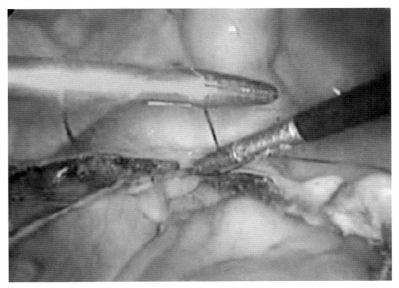

FIGURE 5.100: In action

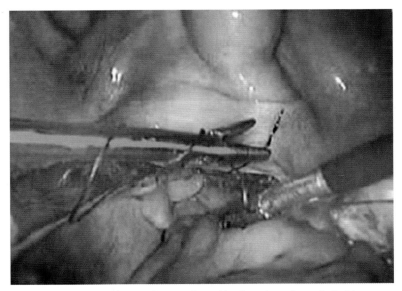

FIGURE 5.101: Role over longer thread in direction of needle holder

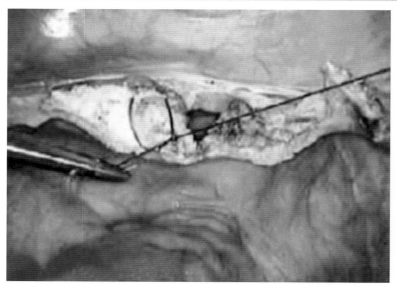

FIGURE 5.102: Tie

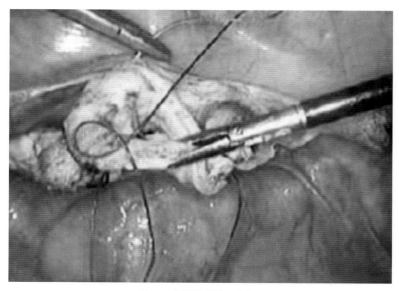

FIGURE 5.103: Other bite

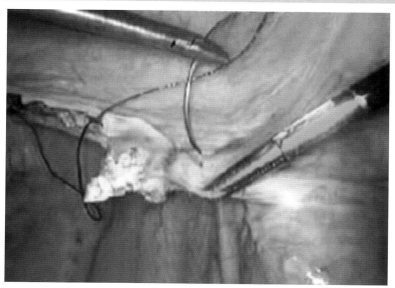

FIGURE 5.104: After vault closer, take stitch from right angle to right round ligament

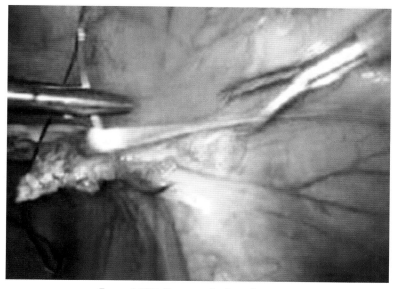

FIGURE 5.105: Pass needle from ligament

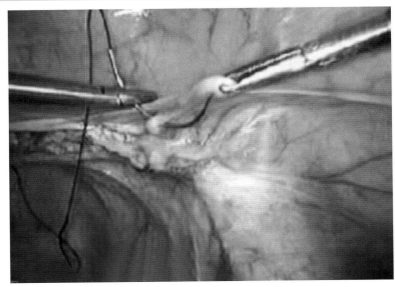

FIGURE 5.106: Again take another bite in round ligament

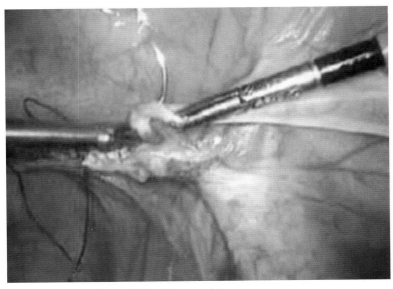

FIGURE 5.107: Adequate bites are necessary

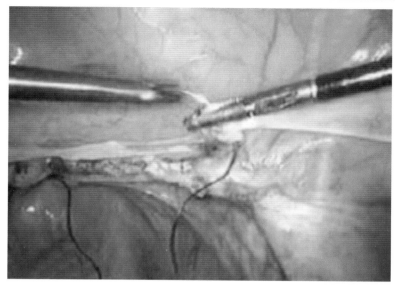

FIGURE **5.108:** Pass needle

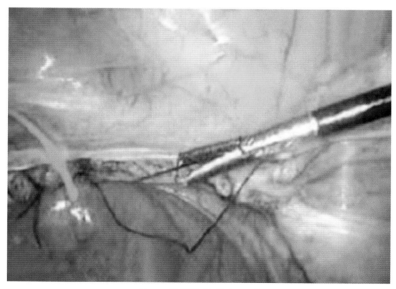

FIGURE **5.109:** Pull thread

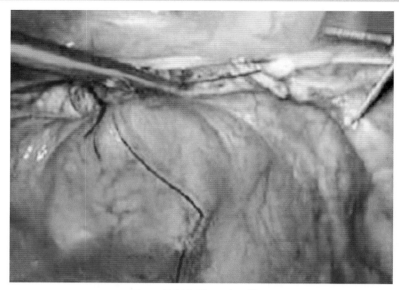

FIGURE 5.110: Thread pulling

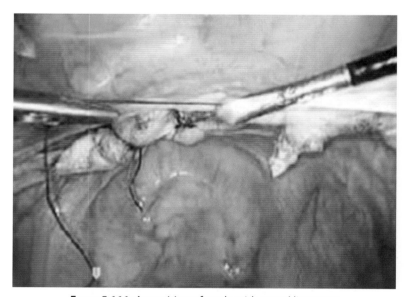

FIGURE 5.111: Apposition of angle with round ligament

- Vault become higher level while pulling thread
- Uterosacral, round ligament and cardinal comes together
- It brings normal anatomical support.

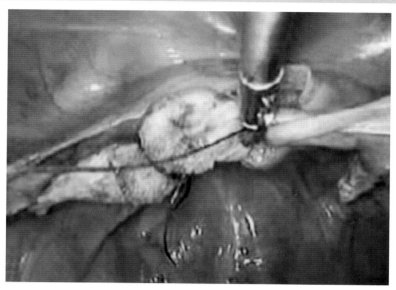

FIGURE 5.112: Come closer all ligament

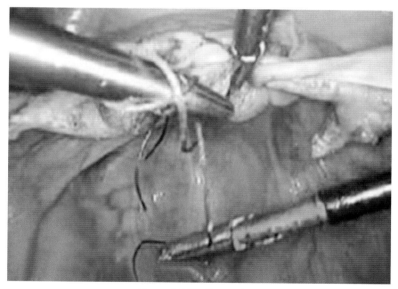

FIGURE 5.113: Knot tying

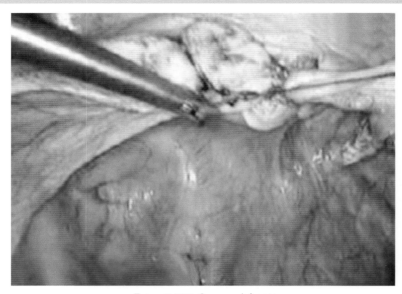

FIGURE 5.114: Surgeon's knot

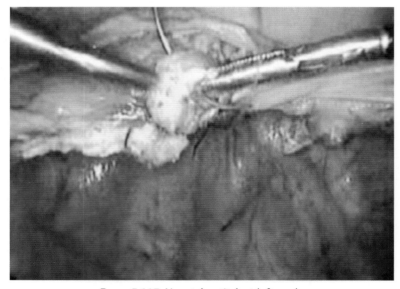

FIGURE 5.115: Now take stitch at left angle

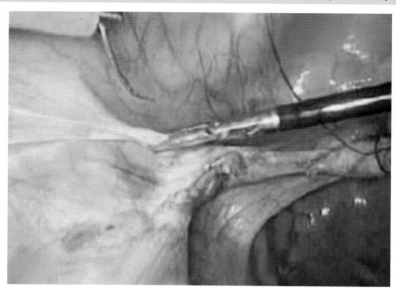

FIGURE 5.116: Then stitch on left round ligament

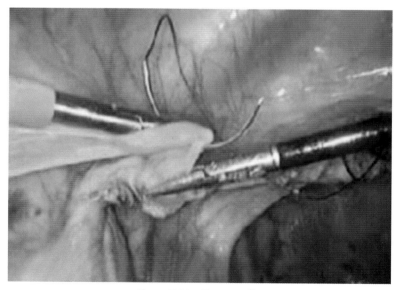

FIGURE 5.117: Pass needle

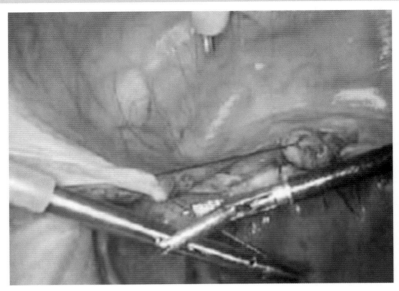

FIGURE 5.118: Pull threads

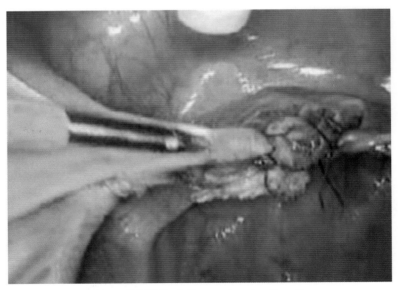

FIGURE 5.119: Push ligament and pull vault

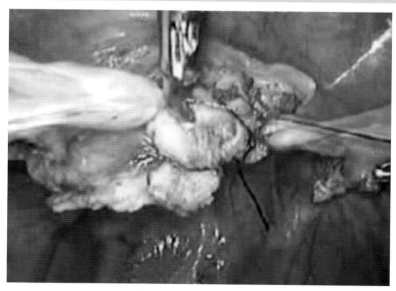

FIGURE 5.120: Knot tying

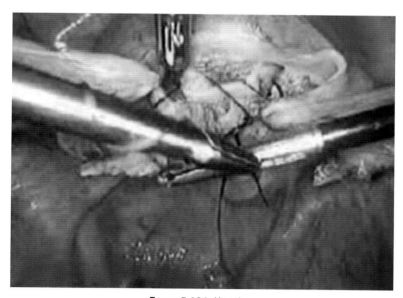

FIGURE 5.121: Knoting

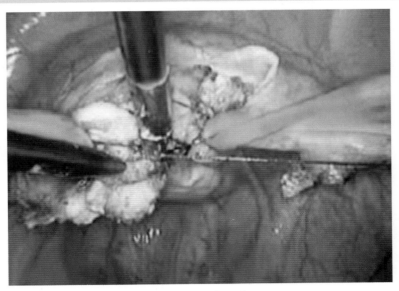

FIGURE 5.122: Last tie

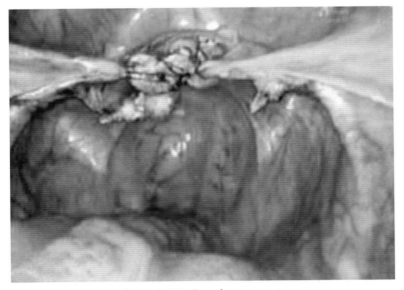

FIGURE 5.123: Complete support

- Final picture
- Vault bring up with all ligaments support.

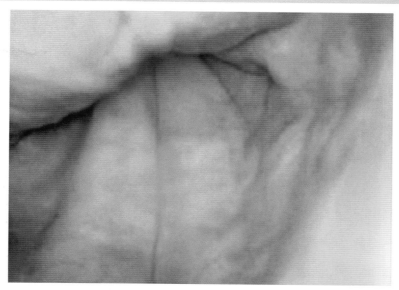

FIGURE 5.124: Vaginal picture

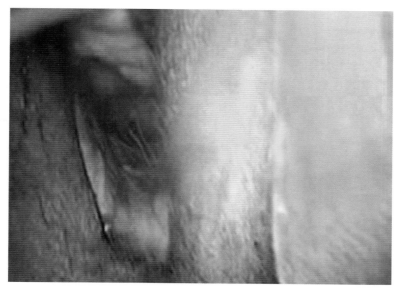

FIGURE 5.125: Vault at higher level

- Everything goes back in normal position
- I did about 88 cases in this way when patient not welling for mesh or poor
- In 2 yrs of fellow up patient does not have any complain.

TOTAL LAPAROSCOPIC HYSTERECTOMY IN CASE OF BROAD LIGAMENT FIBROID

Case-10

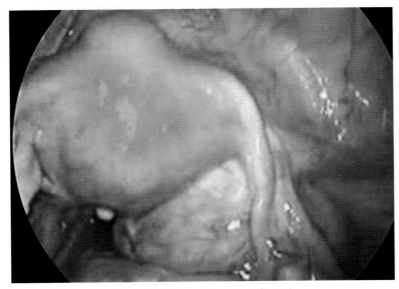

FIGURE 5.126: Broad ligament fibroid

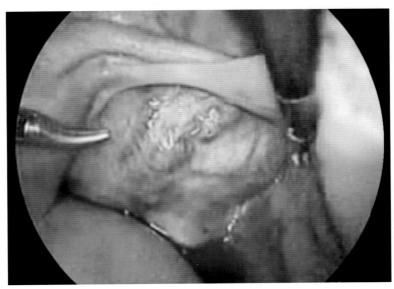

FIGURE 5.127: Ureter close to fibroid

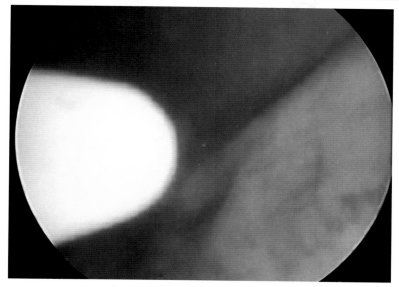

FIGURE 5.128: Cystoscopic stenting of right ureter

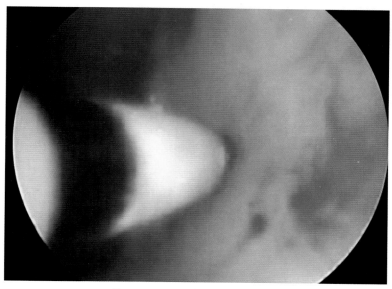

FIGURE 5.129: Right ureteric orifice

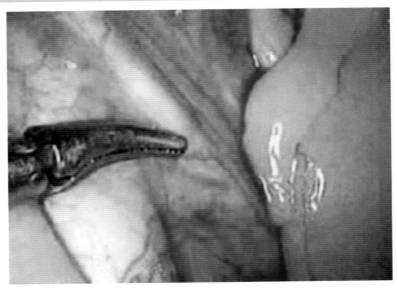

Figure 5.130: Ureter with stent

- Isolation of right ureter by sent
- Then begin with surgery.

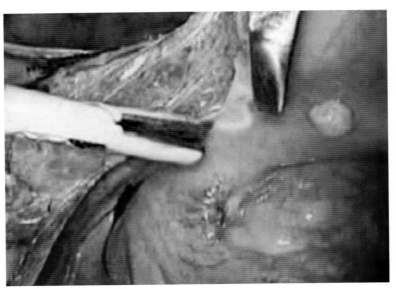

Figure 5.131: Left side dissection

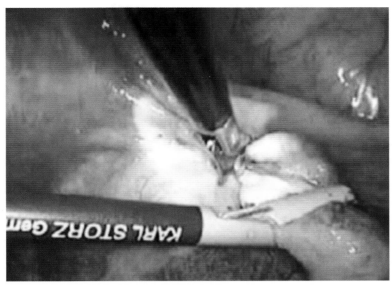

FIGURE 5.132: Right side dissection

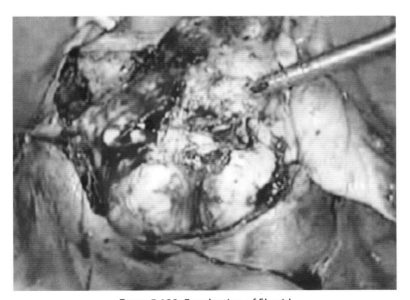

FIGURE 5.133: Enucleation of fibroid

- After both cornual, left uterine and bladder dissection then go for myoma removal
- Right side uterine is below fibroid
- Then tackle right uterine and ligaments.

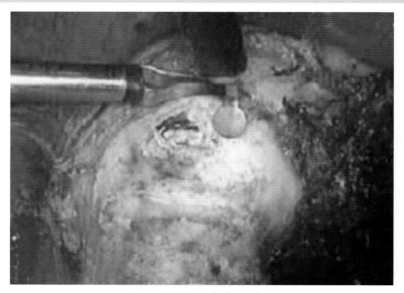

FIGURE 5.134: Vault dissection

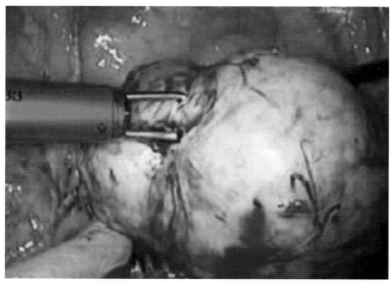

FIGURE 5.135: Morcellation of myoma

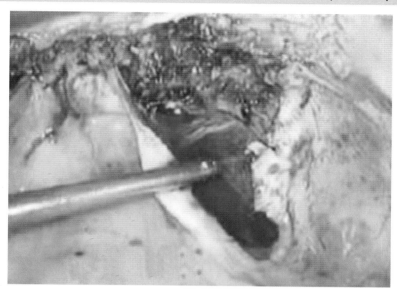

FIGURE 5.136: End of surgery

RADHE TECHNIQUE OF PRIMARY PORT ENTRY

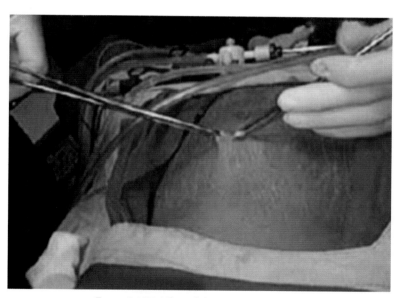

FIGURE 5.137: Lift umbilicus at center point

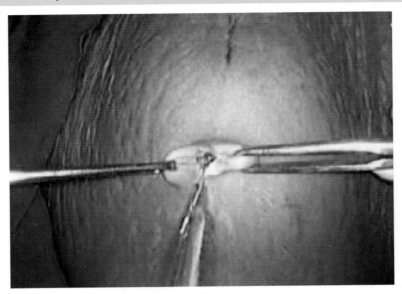

FIGURE 5.138: Cut skin at center point

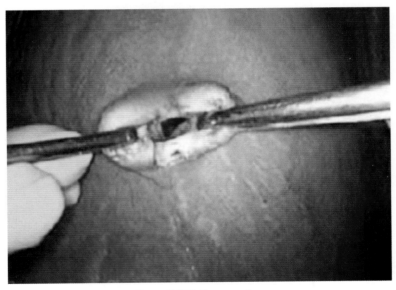

FIGURE 5.139: See opening

- Cutting of sheath
- Peritoneum may open.

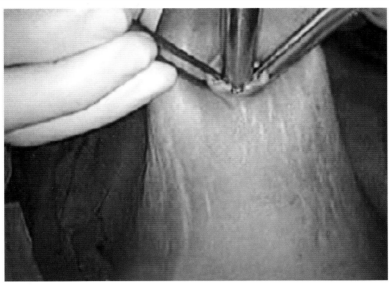

FIGURE 5.140: Trocar insertion

- Primary port entry
- Lift abdominal wall and insert trocar.

SECONDARY PORTS INSERTION

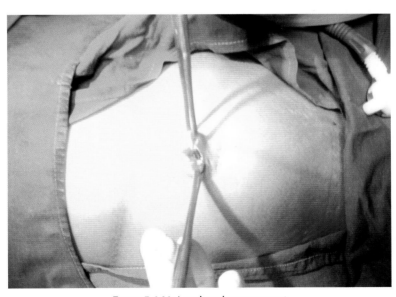

FIGURE 5.141: Landmark assessment

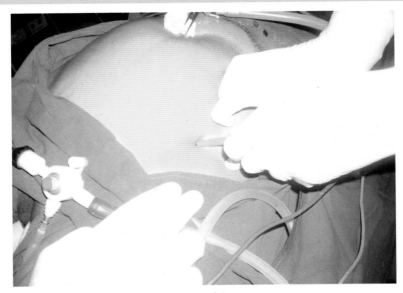

FIGURE **5.142:** Left lower port

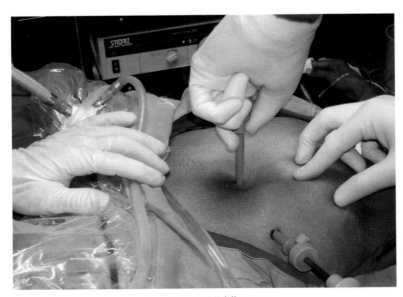

FIGURE **5.143:** Middle port

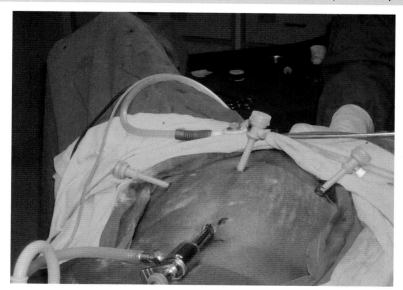

FIGURE 5.144: Right lower port

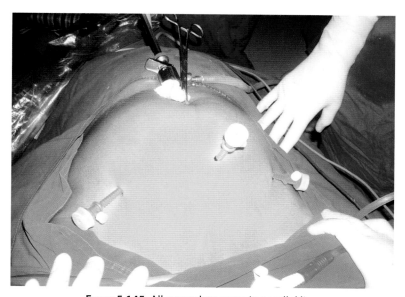

FIGURE 5.145: All secondary ports in parallel line

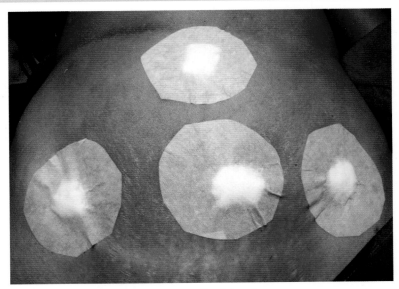

FIGURE 5.146: Final dressing

CHAPTER

6

Difficulties During Total Laparoscopic Hysterectomy

We will discuss only problems while performing Laparoscopic Hysterectomy.

Bleeding at Any Stage of Surgery

Steps to prevent bleeding are following:
- Proper coagulation is must
- Give intermittent of current rather than constant current
- Understand sign of coagulation
- Stoppage of bubble
- Change of tissue colors from Red-White-yellow, coagulation over .If we do more than charring happen and forceps also stuck with tissue
- More coagulation and less cut
- Coagulate and cut rather than cut and coagulate.

Difficulties in Dissection

- Proper manipulation of uterus with Sukhadiya's Manipulator.
- Principal of cutting—stretch any part properly, it can cut very easily.

CHAPTER
7
Complications of Total Laparoscopic Hysterectomy

Fewer the case load, more the complication rate.

Complications can be related to:

a. Anesthesia
b. Access
c. Patient
d. Procedure
e. Position
f. Instrument.

- As such, no major complications with TLH if, you have done procedure properly
- But any procedure have its own complication if activity not done in right way
- Take care of three Bs like:
    1. Bowel
    2. Bladder
    3. Bleeding.
- I have following complications in TLH
    – Bladder injury:
        - A case of frozen abdomen is that everything completely adherent.
        - While dissection, bladder was open and close in two layer.

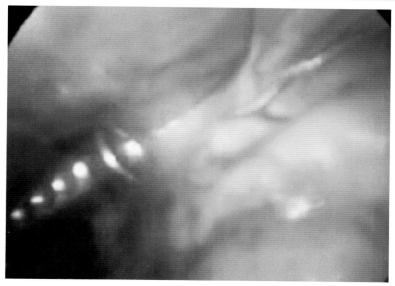

FIGURE 7.1: Frozen abdomen

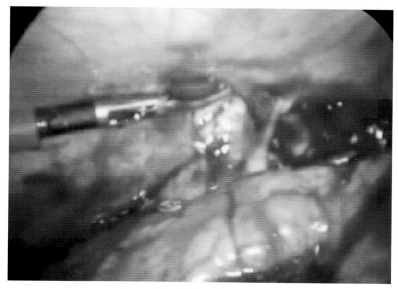

FIGURE 7.2: Adhesiolysis started

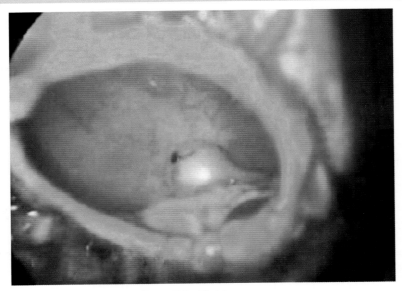

FIGURE 7.3: Bladder open

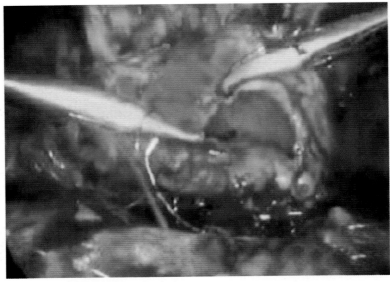

FIGURE 7.4: Close bladder in two layers with 3-0 centicryl

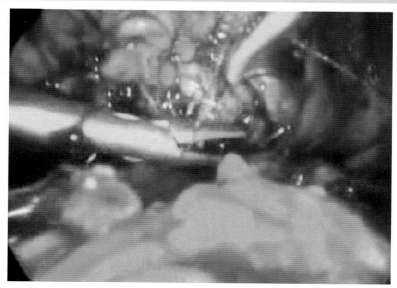

FIGURE 7.5: After complete closer start TLH and finish procedure

Ureteric Injury

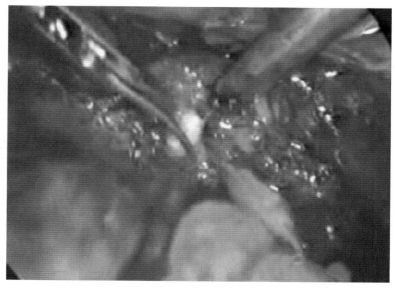

FIGURE 7.6: Sharp cut on right ureter

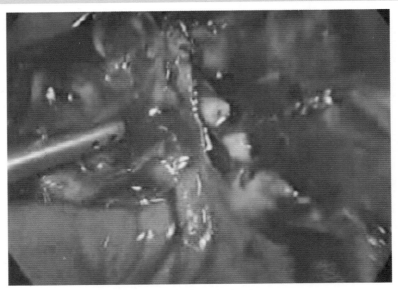

FIGURE 7.7: Both ends clearly seen

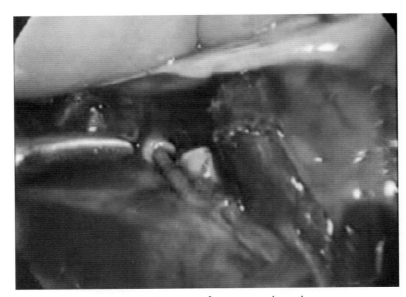

FIGURE 7.8: Stent pass from one end to other

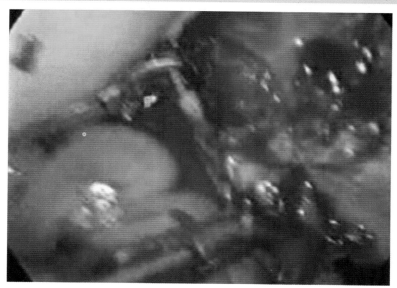

FIGURE 7.9: Stent passed

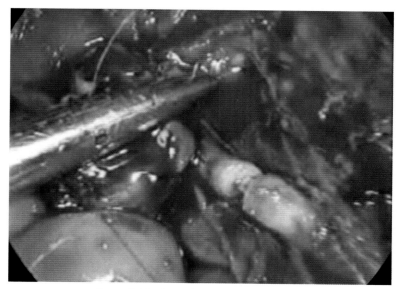

FIGURE 7.10: Start closer with 6-0 centicryl

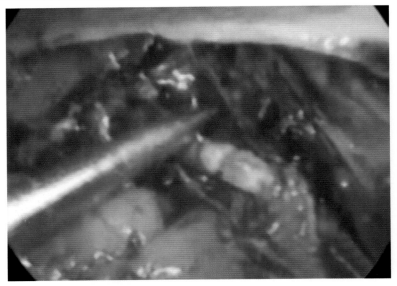

FIGURE 7.11: Second stitch taken

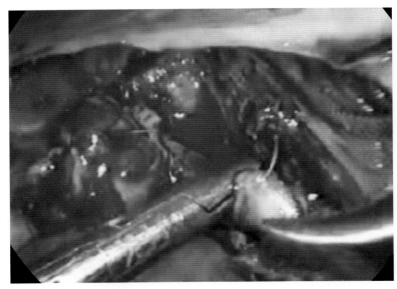

FIGURE 7.12: Needle passes to opposite end

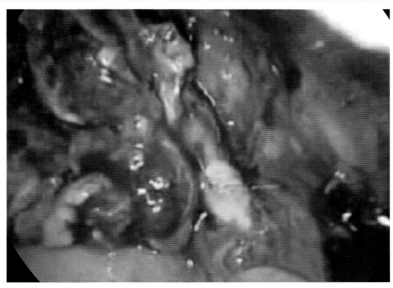

FIGURE 7.13: Suturing over

Umbilical Hernia Repair

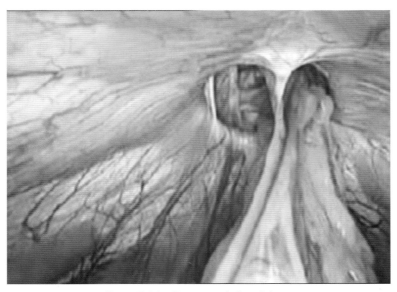

FIGURE 7.14: Omentum in hernial sac

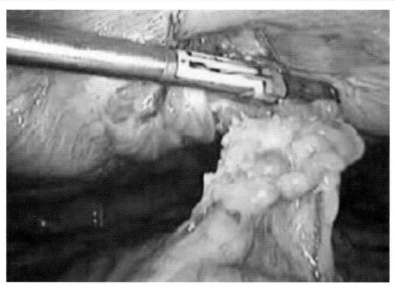

FIGURE 7.15: Dissection of omentum from sac

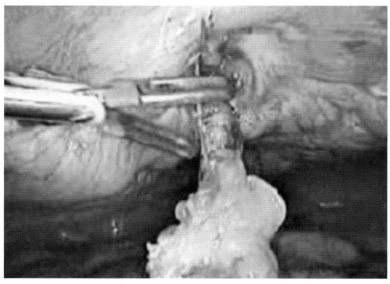

FIGURE 7.16: Completely empty sac before closer to sac

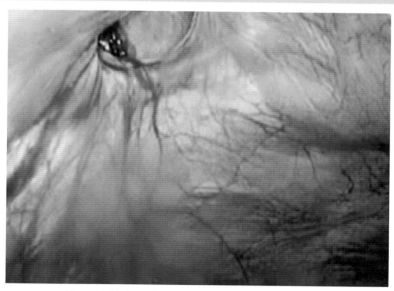

FIGURE 7.17: Now hernial defect ready for meshplasty

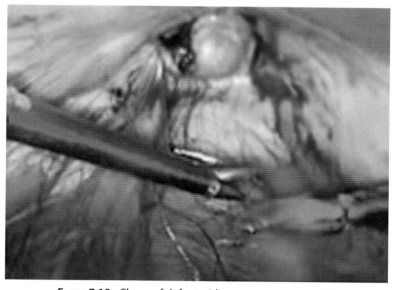

FIGURE 7.18: Closer of defect with gortex suture material

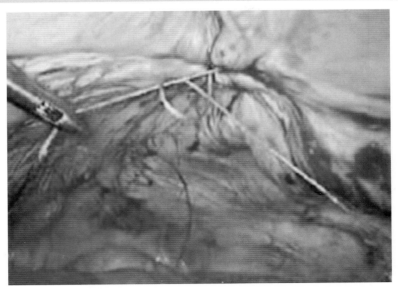

FIGURE 7.19: Purse string

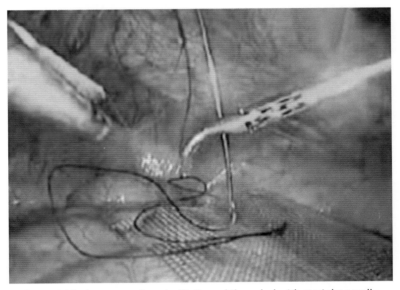

FIGURE 7.20: In center of mesh silk tie and threaded with straight needle

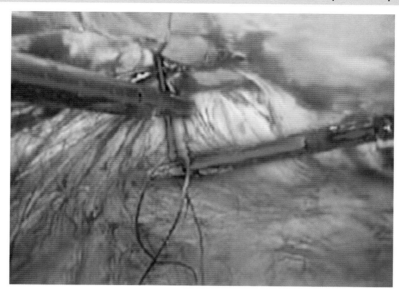

FIGURE 7.21: Passage of needle through gap

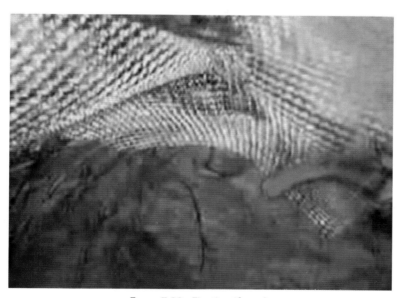

FIGURE 7.22: Fixation if mesh

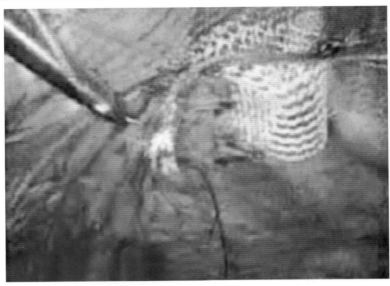

FIGURE 7.23: Mesh fix to abdominal wall with intermittent stitch

CHAPTER
8
How to Use Sukhadiya's Manipulator

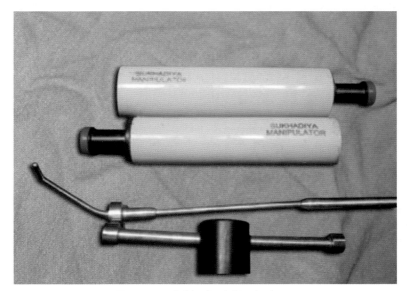

FIGURE **8.1:** Sukhadiya's Manipulator

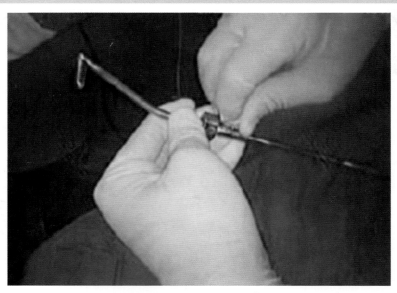

Figure 8.2: Measurement of UCL

HOW DO FIX SUKHADIYA'S MANIPULATOR?

Three parts:
1. Fixation of rod
2. Passage of tube
3. Manipulation.

1. *Fixation of rod:* Measurement of UCL then accordingly passes rod in uterine cavity. After taking stitch on anterior and posterior lip of cervix to fix rod.
2. Then pass tube over rod and fix handle for better movement.
3. While working on left side of uterus move uterus towards right side. When we go towards uterine then you should push uterus upward. Same way for opposite side. For vault dissection push tube so, it make vault more prominent. At a time just pull of rod outside.

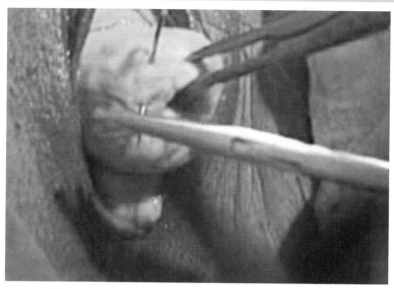

FIGURE 8.3: First stitch on right side of anterior cervical lip

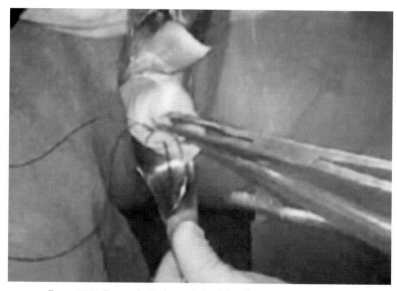

FIGURE 8.4: Second stitch on right side of posterior cervical lip

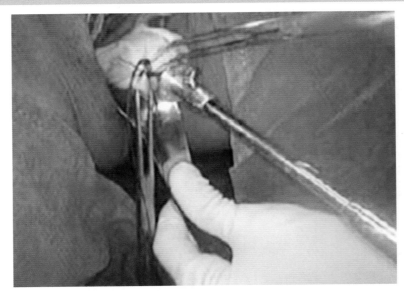

FIGURE 8.5: Then tie

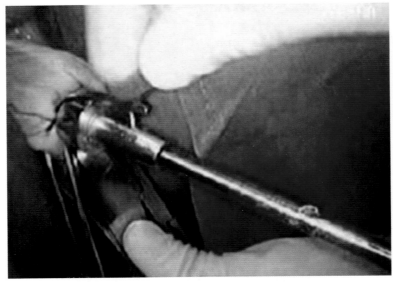

FIGURE 8.6: Fix thread on the screw

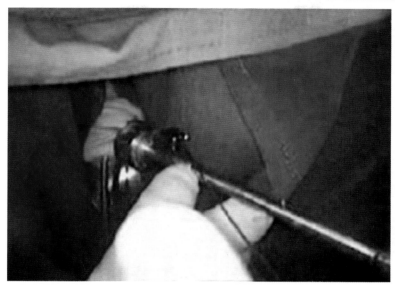

FIGURE 8.7: Scrolling of thread

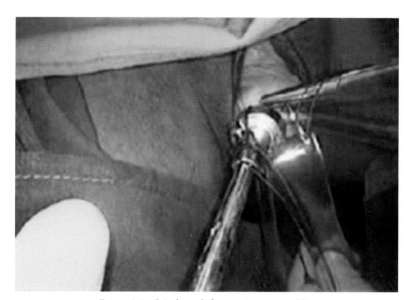

FIGURE 8.8: Stitch on left anterior cervical lip

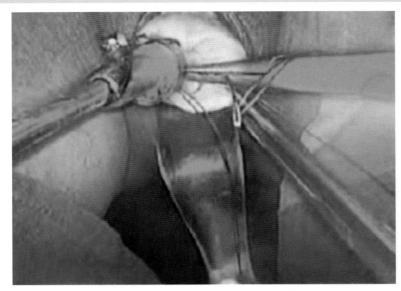

FIGURE 8.9: Stitch on posterior cervical lip

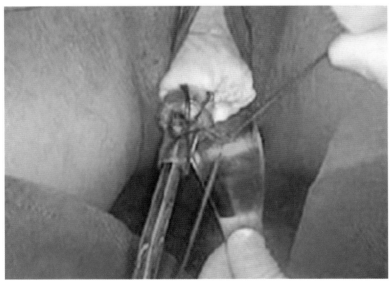

FIGURE 8.10: Lastly tie

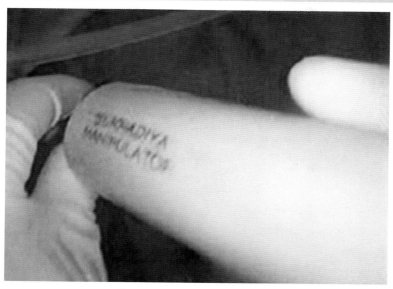

FIGURE 8.11: Pass tube over rod

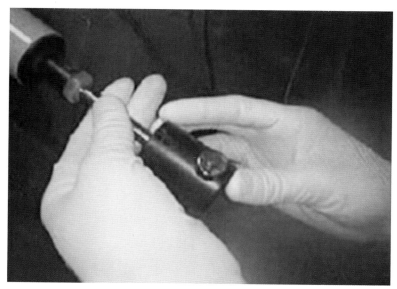

FIGURE 8.12: Fix handle

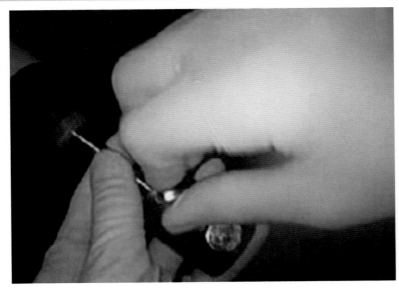

FIGURE 8.13: Manipulator is fix and ready for use

C H A P T E R

Role of Anesthesia

ANESTHESIA AND LAPAROSCOPY

Introduction

Laparoscopy is insufflation of CO_2 in peritoneal cavity under controlled pressure and it causes increase in intra-abdominal pressure (IAP).

Pathophysiology

1. Initially CO_2 insufflation in peritoneal cavity causes stretching of peritoneum and some times bradycardia
2. Rise in IAP reduces lung volumes and increase in pulmonary resistance.
3. Absorption of CO_2 from peritoneum causes hypercarbia and which causes stress response to cardiovascular system, which ultimately leads to hypertension and tachycardia.
4. Rise in IAP can cause fall in cardiac output in compromise patients.
5. Increase in IAP may reduce lower esophageal sphincter tone and risk of regurgitation of gastric content increases.
6. Head low position increases intracranial pressure, intraocular pressure and increase in risk of regurgitation.

To overcome the above pathophysiological changes, patient must be under general anesthesia and controlled mechanical ventilation with closed. Circuit and nasogastric tube in position after induction with basic monitoring: SpO2, ECG, NIBP, and ETCO2.

Anesthesia Protocol for Laparoscopy Surgery

IV Drip : RL 1 Lit.

Preoperative : Inj Gylcopyrolate 1 amp.
Inj Ranitidine 1 amp
Inj Tramadol 50 mg or Inj Fentanyl 50 mcg IV slowly

Induction : Preoxygenation
Inj Thiopental 8 mg/kg + Inj Scoline 2 mg/kg
After intubation-Inj Diclofenac 1 amp IM

Maintenance : O_2 + N_2O + Inj Propofol 6-10 mg/kg/min
OR Isofyrane + Inj Vecuronium of Inj Atracurium
For BP control- Inj Nitroglyrine if required
At the end of surgery Inj Sensorcaine at port site (Local Infiltration)

Reversal	:	Inj Myopyrolate 5 ml IV
		Inj Emeset 4 ml IV
		Inj Tramadol 50 mg IV slowly
Postoperative	:	O_2 with nasal cannula for 1 hour.
Remarks	:	Close circuit (with soda lime) helps in blood pressure control
		By removing CO_2 from expiration and save gases.

Dr Vishnu Patel
MD Anesth
Mehsana

CHAPTER
10

Advantages of Total Laparoscopic Hysterectomy

- We all know TLH has its own real advantage, no one can replace it.
- It is true laparoscopic approach
- It is intrafascial hysterectomy
- Avoiding injury to ligaments and maintaining vascularity and innervation of the Pelvic tissue
- Less chance of bladder, ureter and less surgical trauma
- Vault support is maintained and vaginal length is not shortening or tenting
- Vault closure does not cause inversion of vaginal mucosa so, less chances of vault granulation
- Intact pericervical ring so, prevents postoperative vault prolapse and maintain good innervation
- With pelvic floor repair procedures easy to carry out
- Our experience of more than 5400 TLH.

11 FOGSI Recognized Radhe Endoscopy Training Centre

- Our Centre is FOGSI Recognized Endoscopy Training Centre
  - Normally, we organize every 3-monthly training courses in February, July and November
  - But according to requirement we also arrange courses every monthly
  - In each course kept minimum 30-35 cases
  - We have different pelvic trainer modules
  - Arrangement of special endosuturing session
  - Allow candidate hand on training
  - Different lectures
  - Video presentation
  - Training kids
  - Theory material (Endo easy booklet)
  - Video library of all variety of laparoscopic surgeries
  - Exhalent follow-up in future
  - Proper guidance related to laparoscopy
  - Build up confidence and remove fear.

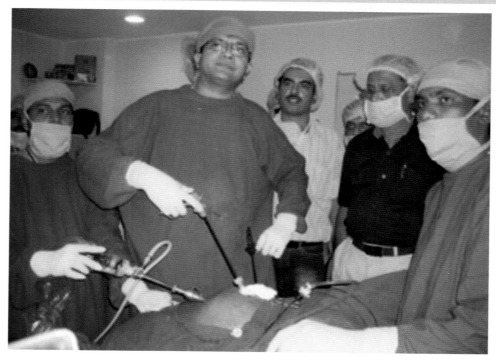

FIGURE 11.1: Live presentation

• Laparoscopy in progress

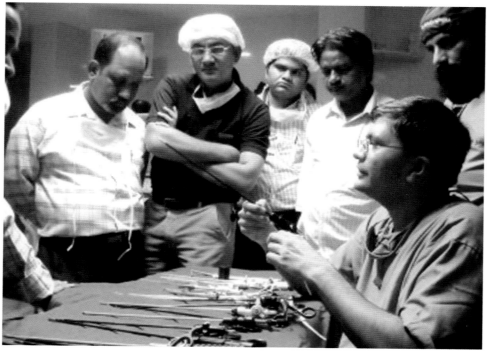

FIGURE 11.2: Lectures

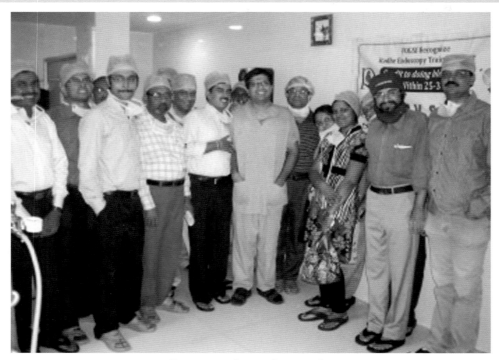

FIGURE **11.3:** Group photography

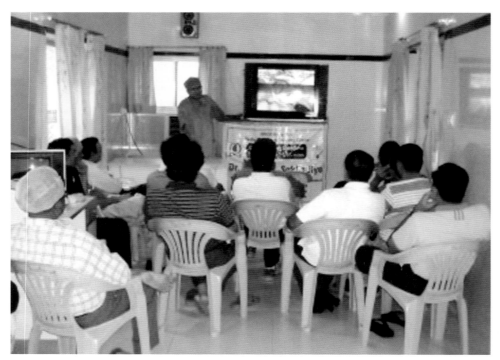

FIGURE **11.4:** Video presentation

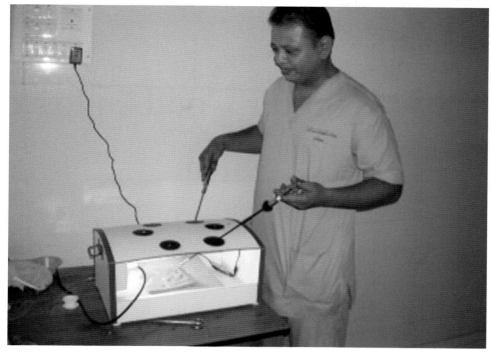

FIGURE 11.5: Pelvic trainer

CHAPTER
12   Tip for Good Endoscopist

1. First, become a good human being.
2. Cool and calm while working.
3. Understand limitation:
   - Our
   - Staff
   - Some technical.
4. Laparoscopy orientation.
5. Pray to God.

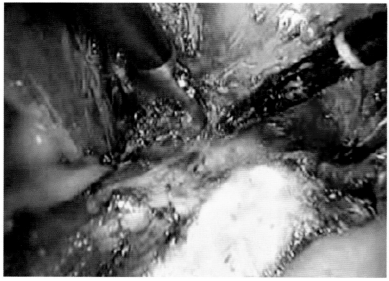

FIGURE 12.1: Pelvic trainer

Index